Therapeutic Aesthetics

RADICAL AESTHETICS – RADICAL ART

Series editors: Jane Tormey and Gillian Whiteley
(Loughborough University, UK)

Promoting debate, confronting conventions and formulating alternative ways of thinking, Jane Tormey and Gillian Whiteley explore what radical aesthetics might mean in the twenty-first century. This new books series, *Radical Aesthetics – Radical Art* (*RaRa*), reconsiders the relationship between how art is practised and how art is theorized. Striving to liberate theories of aesthetics from visual traditions, this series of single-authored titles expands the parameters of art and aesthetics in a creative and meaningful way. Encompassing the multisensory, collaborative, participatory and transitory practices that have developed over the last twenty years, *Radical Aesthetics – Radical Art* is an innovative and revolutionary take on the intersection between theory and practice.

Published and forthcoming in the series:

Practical Aesthetics: Events, Affects and Art after 9/11, Jill Bennett

Transitional Aesthetics: Contemporary Art at the Edge of Europe, Uros Cvoro

Eco-Aesthetics: Art, Literature and Architecture in a Period of Climate Change, Malcolm Miles

Civic Aesthetics: Militarism in Israeli Art and Visual Culture, Noa Roei

Counter-Memorial Aesthetics: Refugees, Contemporary Art and the Politics of Memory, Veronica Tello

Working Aesthetics: Labour, Art and Capitalism, Danielle Child

Art, Politics and the Pamphleteer, edited by Jane Tormey and Gillian Whiteley

For further information or enquiries please contact *RaRa* series editors:
Jane Tormey: j.tormey@lboro.ac.uk
Gillian Whiteley: g.whiteley@lboro.ac.uk

Therapeutic Aesthetics:

Performative Encounters in Moving Image Artworks

Maria Walsh

BLOOMSBURY ACADEMIC
LONDON • NEW YORK • OXFORD • NEW DELHI • SYDNEY

BLOOMSBURY ACADEMIC
Bloomsbury Publishing Plc
50 Bedford Square, London, WC1B 3DP, UK
1385 Broadway, New York, NY 10018, USA

BLOOMSBURY, BLOOMSBURY ACADEMIC and the Diana logo
are trademarks of Bloomsbury Publishing Plc

First published in Great Britain 2021

Cover image: *Primal Speech*, installation by Liz Magic Laser (2016), from the exhibition
Psyche als Schauplatz des Politischen (Psyche as the Scene of the Political) at Staatliche
Kunsthalle Baden-Baden, Germany
(© Uli Deck / DPA / Alamy Live News)

A catalogue record for this book is available from the British Library.

Library of Congress Cataloging-in-Publication Data
Names: Walsh, Maria, author.
Title: Therapeutic aesthetics : performative encounters in moving
image artworks / Maria Walsh.
Description: London ; New York : Bloomsbury Academic, 2021. |
Series: Radical aesthetics-radical art | Includes bibliographical references and index.
Identifiers: LCCN 2020029960 | ISBN 9781350093157 (hardback) | ISBN 9781350189430
(paperback) | ISBN 9781350093133 (ebook) | ISBN 9781350093140 (epub)
Subjects: LCSH: Art therapy.
Classification: LCC RC489.A7 W37 2021 | DDC 615.8/5156–dc23
LC record available at https://lccn.loc.gov/2020029960

ISBN: HB: 978-1-3500-9315-7
ePDF: 978-1-3500-9313-3
eBook: 978-1-3500-9314-0

Series: Radical Aesthetics-Radical Art (RARA)

Typeset by Integra Software Services Pvt. Ltd.

To find out more about our authors and books visit www.bloomsbury.com
and sign up for our newsletters.

Contents

List of Figures		vi
Preface		viii
Acknowledgements		x
1	Introduction	1
2	Setting the scene – two supplementary vignettes	17
3	The imbrication of poison and cure in Harun Farocki	27
4	Homeopathic mimicry in Omer Fast's war trilogy	47
5	Melanie Gilligan's signifying semiologies and the micro-resistance of collective subjectivity	67
6	Pharmacological reparation in Liz Magic Laser's *Primal Speech*	87
7	Leigh Ledare's pharmacological aesthetics of group analysis	107
8	Aesthetic modes of performative truth-telling in *The O Show* and *Self Made*	127
9	The transitional pleasures of emotional labour in Lucy Beech's and Rehana Zaman's videos	151
10	Conclusion: Toxicity and self-care – two poles of pharmacological aesthetics	171
Notes		185
Bibliography		206
Index		222

List of Figures

2.1 Pipilotti Rist, *Worry Will Vanish*, 2014. © Pipilotti Rist. Courtesy the artist, Hauser & Wirth and Luhring Augustine 18

3.1 Harun Farocki, *Serious Games (I–IV)*, 2010. Serious Games I: Watson Is Down, Video (colour, sound) 8 min. Courtesy HARUN FAROCKI FILMPRODUKTION and Greene Naftali, New York 37

3.2 Harun Farocki, *Serious Games (I–IV)*, 2010. Serious Games III: Immersion (2009), Video (colour, sound) 20 min. Courtesy HARUN FAROCKI FILMPRODUKTION and Greene Naftali, New York 38

3.3 Harun Farocki, *Serious Games (I–IV)*, 2010. Serious Games IV: A Sun With No Shadow, Video (colour, sound). Courtesy HARUN FAROCKI FILMPRODUKTION and Greene Naftali, New York 41

4.1 Omer Fast, *The Casting*, 2007. Four-channel video installation, colour, sound, duration: 14 minutes, Credit: Nick Trikonis, Courtesy of the artist and James Cohan, New York 51

4.2 Omer Fast, *The Casting* 2007. Four-channel video installation, colour, sound. Duration: 14 minutes, Credit: Nick Trikonis, Courtesy of the artist and James Cohan, New York 52

4.3 Krzysztof Wodiczko, *Abraham Lincoln: War Veteran Projection, Union Square, New York*, 2012. © Krzysztof Wodiczko. Courtesy Galerie Lelong & Co., New York 57

4.4 Omer Fast, *5000 Feet is the Best*, 2011. Single channel HD video, colour, sound. Duration: 30 minutes looped, Credit: Nick Trikonis, Courtesy of the artist and James Cohan, New York 61

5.1 Melanie Gilligan, *Popular Unrest*, 2010; Courtesy the artist and Galerie Max Mayer, Düsseldorf 74

5.2 Melanie Gilligan, *The Common Sense*, 2014; Courtesy the artist and Galerie Max Mayer, Düsseldorf 84

6.1 Liz Magic Laser, *I Feel Your Pain* (2011), Production Still by Yola Monakhov, Courtesy of the artist 91
6.2 Liz Magic Laser, *Primal Speech* (2016), video still, Courtesy of the artist 99
7.1 Leigh Ledare *The Large Group (Zurich)*, 2016. Courtesy of the artist 115
7.2 Leigh Ledare *The Large Group (Zurich)*, 2016. Courtesy of the artist 115
7.3 Leigh Ledare *The Task*, 2017. Courtesy of the artist 121
8.1 Oriana Fox, *The O Show: The Therapeutic Potential of Performance*, 2012. (video still) Courtesy of the artist 131
8.2 Oriana Fox, *The O Show: You're Only as Sick as Your Secrets*, 2019. (production still) Courtesy of the artist and Block 336 138
8.3 Gillian Wearing *Self Made* (2010) colour film with sound, 84 minutes. © Gillian Wearing, courtesy Maureen Paley, London 143
8.4 Gillian Wearing *Self Made* (2010) colour film with sound, 84 minutes. © Gillian Wearing, courtesy Maureen Paley, London 144
9.1 Lucy Beech, *Cannibals*, 2013. Video still. Courtesy of the artist 158
9.2 Rehana Zaman, *Some Women, Other Women and All the Bittermen*, 2014. Video still. Courtesy of the artist 168
10.1 Rehana Zaman, *Sharla Shabana Sojourner Selena*, 2016. Video still. Courtesy of the artist 180

Preface

The *RaRa* series explores what aesthetics might mean in the twenty-first century by integrating practice and theory and firmly embedding the discussion of artworks in the social. Maria Walsh's *Therapeutic Aesthetics* contributes a focused analysis of a range of contemporary artists' practices from the perspective of contemporary psychoanalytical and political theories, with particular reference to film and video. Making a clear distinction between 'art therapy' and the therapeutic tropes and discourses deployed as both subject matter and form within these moving image art practices, the book makes a unique contribution to our series as it provides a new context for radicality and the intersection of art, aesthetics and politics.

Walsh traces a cultural 'turn' to therapeutic discourse, finding evidence in a range of narratives to do with psychological disorders such as post-traumatic stress disorder, anxiety, burn-out and depression. Furthermore, she identifies how therapeutic form is invoked by artists' films that model themselves on therapy scenarios, often involving the artist as a pseudo-therapist or interviewer. She argues that moving image artworks, in particular, frequently instigate a *faux* therapeutic encounter through their performance of the kind of interpretive processes of experience usually associated with psychoanalysis. Deploying the motif of the pharmacological as both remedy and poison, she highlights the politicized role and impact of these strategies, arguing that these forms of practice allow viewers to acknowledge, rather than heal, the psychical disturbances and traumas of emotional life under cognitive capitalism. Ultimately, Walsh's book offers an exploration of the problematic aspects of therapeutic practices, but it also posits hope for the contribution that art practices make in helping us see and experience how our desires and emotions can be harnessed to make social change rather than for the exploitative instrumentalization of cognitive capitalism.

Therapeutic Aesthetics: Performative Encounters in Moving Image Artworks provides a series of important case studies for artists, researchers and students in the field of contemporary art history, cultural studies, film and media and performance studies. This study is timely in its contribution and response to the affective aspects of lived experience under contemporary capitalism. As such, the book's concerns lie very much within the territory of the *RaRa* series and it makes a significant addition to the range of current titles that address some of the most pressing issues of our time.

RaRa series editors
Jane Tormey and Gillian Whiteley
April 2020

Acknowledgements

I would like to thank my commissioning editor Liza Thompson for her enthusiasm for this project when I initially approached Bloomsbury with my proposal. Thanks also to the editors of the Radical Aesthetics series, Jane Tormey and Gillian Whiteley, for accepting my book in this series and to the anonymous peer reviewers who gave feedback on my proposal and manuscript.

I would like to acknowledge the support of the University of the Arts London Research Management Group who granted me sabbatical leave so that I could bring my research for this book to fruition. A special thanks to my colleague Dr Rosa Nogués, who assisted me with my bibliographic references in the final stages of writing.

Preliminary and/or related research was presented at various symposia and conferences: aspects of Chapters 3 and 4 were presented at the 'Technologies of Romance' symposium at the Whitechapel Gallery Auditorium on 5 March 2017 and at the annual Film-Philosophy conference at Lancaster University on 5 July 2017. Thanks to Paul O'Kane for inviting me to present my research at the former event. Parts of Chapter 8 were included in a public lecture 'Performative Therapeutics in Contemporary Artists' Moving Image' at Jerwood Space on 19 February 2018. Thanks to Lauren Houlton for this invitation.

Related research on trauma was presented at the 'Performance, Trauma and Victimhood' symposium at UCL on 13 June 2018, while preliminary research for Chapter 10 was presented at the Iniva Research Network: Duties of Self-Care at Shoreditch Town Hall on 25 October 2018. Thanks to everyone who hosted these platforms. Thanks also to Patricia Bickers, editor of *Art Monthly*, for commissioning a feature based on nothing more than my professed interest in Liz Magic Laser's *Primal Speech*. Writing 'Art: A Suitable Case for Treatment?' *Art Monthly* 415: April 2018, pp.14–17 helped consolidate ideas.

An earlier version of Chapter 8, 'Acts of Laughter, Acts of Tears: The Production of "Truth-Effects"' in Oriana Fox's *The O Show* and Gillian

Wearing's *Self Made*, was published in *NECSUS: European Journal of Media Studies*, eds. Ilona Hongisto, Toni Pape and Alanna Thain, http://www.necsus-ejms.org/acts-of-laughter-acts-of-tears-the-production-of-truth-effects-in-oriana-foxs-the-o-show-and-gillian-wearings-self-made/, accessed 6 June 2017. The updated version in this book is published with kind permission of Amsterdam University Press. I would particularly like to thank the anonymous peer reviewers of this earlier article for their rigorous, yet supportive, critiques which gave me confidence that my counterintuitive idea was worth pursuing. An earlier version of Chapter 9, 'Female Solidarity as Uncommodified Value: Lucy Beech's *Cannibals*, and Rehana Zaman's *Some Women, Other Women and All the Bittermen*', was published in *Women Artists, Feminism and the Moving Image*, ed. Lucy Reynolds, London and New York: Bloomsbury, 2019. I would like to thank Lucy Reynolds for her generous invitation to contribute to this book without imposing any strictures other than word length. My updated version of that earlier chapter is published here with kind permission of Bloomsbury. I would also like to thank other colleagues involved in the journal *MIRAJ*, especially Cate Elwes, who invited me to co-edit the *Feminisms* special issue with her in 2014; my research for my article in that edition feeding indirectly into the final chapters of this book.

Very special thanks to the artists and galleries who provided images *gratis*. This was very welcome in the current climate.

I am grateful to the artists, academics and critics whose work has inspired this book and, unwittingly, enabled me to 'use' it in the Winnicottian sense. In this spirit, I dedicate this book to its potential users.

1

Introduction

This book is motivated by what might seem, at first, to be a counterintuitive idea: that is, that therapeutic aesthetics necessarily involves both toxicity and cure.[1] Usually, the therapeutic is thought of in relation to healing, its meaning being to treat medicinally, to cure. However, treatment, whether by drugs or alternative medicine, including the psy therapies, could be said to be inherently pharmacological. That is to say that the pharmacological, as I derive it from the ancient Greek term 'pharmakon', is a treatment that is both a poison and a remedy. While in common parlance every drug is considered to have side effects, my argument will err more on the side of the nonseparability of the beneficent and the harmful. Discussing a selective number of moving image artworks in the chapters that follow, I shall show how the philosophical ambivalence of the 'pharmakon' is echoed in their conflictual performances of art treatments.

Aesthetics too, in its association with beauty and sensory experience, is usually considered somewhat remedial, so it would seem counterintuitive to pair aesthetics with the ambivalence of the pharmacological.[2] However, aside from the sense that, in Western art practice since at least the 1960s, beauty in art appears outmoded,[3] in a technologically mediated environment, the terms of aesthetic analysis have shifted to focus on 'media dynamics, affect and perception' as well as being 'informed by and derived from practical, real-world encounters' (Bennett, 2012: 2). The 'real-world encounter' that provides a model for the moving image artworks that I discuss in this book is a loosely articulated therapeutic scenario in which speaking is used as a treatment. This treatment, including narrative and performative modes of address, is not only inherently pharmacological, but, being embedded in a neoliberal socio-economic order that I refer to as cognitive capitalism, it is necessarily so. I will have much to say about this order in what follows, but, for now, I simply want to posit that the necessity of situating my moving image case studies in terms of a pharmacological aesthetics has to do with resisting the social proscribing of art as an enhancement of emotional well-being and mental health which is being promulgated by governmental and related institutions in neoliberal capitalism. A pharmacological aesthetics is, I believe, necessary to counter the harnessing of the arts and creativity as instruments for the therapeutic management of subjectivity.

For example in the UK, *The Charter for Arts, Health and Wellbeing*, produced by The National Alliance for Arts, Health & Wellbeing, which launched in 2012, reads: 'The arts, creativity and the imagination are agents of wellness: they help keep the individual resilient, aid recovery and foster a flourishing society.'[4] There is nothing intrinsically wrong with this ethos. However, it is not neutral. Not only are particular, I would say, conservative, forms of cultural and artistic activities promoted, but it is also a way of harnessing the arts to redeem a vanishing welfare state as well as being a means of getting them to justify their usefulness in a climate of reduced public funding. As sociologist Frank Furedi has identified, therapeutic culture, in foregrounding individual emotional needs as the site of social change, acts as a displacement of politics from the public realm and a marginalizing and eclipsing of 'redistributive struggles' (2004: 163). While the politics of 'redistributive struggles' is beyond the scope of my book, of relevance is Furedi's critical account of how in 1990s Britain cultural institutions in general transform their role to become 'centres for therapeutic engagement with excluded people' (Furedi, 2004: 167). This is part of a shift in emphasis from the political management of social problems to the civic responsibility of esteeming the self.[5] In the language of neoliberal capitalism, self-esteem transmogrifies into the promotion of a resilient individual who can survive whatever knocks and blows might be encountered in life without examining the structural reasons for the increase in particular psychopathologies in this climate. To be clear, I am not referring to overtly life-threatening illnesses, but disorders of a psychological nature such as depression, anxiety and exhaustion which, while they may lead to such illnesses, are also manifest as cultural phenomena.[6] In case this statement sounds glib, it may be worth stating that I am no stranger to these symptoms, although, unlike the millennial generation, I have always been resistant to adopting them as personal diagnostic tools. This is not necessarily a moral choice, but due to the fact that my informative years were shaped by a socio-economic order that, although dominated by the toxicity of boom and bust investment, had not yet foreclosed on the future in terms of debt and speculative finance (Berardi, 2011; 2017). Part of the impetus for this book derives from the potential I have found in 'using' moving image to play with and transform, but not heal, such aforementioned symptoms.

The moving image artworks that steer this book are in no way a survey of contemporary artists' works that address the therapeutic per se. Rather, my partly idiosyncratic selection enables me to put forward a particular narrative about the therapeutic as a site of *cultural*, not merely personal, diagnosis and resistance. In this, my case studies are part of a philosophical zeitgeist responding critically to the social, cultural and economic impasses of neoliberal cognitive capitalism. While each chapter mainly focuses on one central case study, this is not to foreground the intentionality of singular artists, but to use their works as tools of analysis that allow me to reflect on pharmacological aesthetics as both a diagnosis of and a micro-resistance to the psychopathologies that emerge within a context of cognitive capitalism. The moving image artworks I stage encounters with range from Omer Fast's loose analogy to 'the talking cure' in his gallery film narratives derived from the symptomatology of veterans' and drone pilots' post-traumatic stress disorder (PTSD) to Oriana Fox's web series chat show which promotes rational emotive behavioural therapy (REBT) as a technique of self-improvement, albeit somewhat ironically. While these two diverse examples are linked, as are all my case studies, by how they variously perform what sociologist Eva Illouz calls a 'therapeutic emotional style' (2008: 15), they also signpost the development of my book's argument from a first part that takes a more overtly diagnostic, critical stance towards the toxic, without denying its remedial potential, to a second half in which the curative dimension of the pharmacological takes the upper hand without denying its toxicity.

Not art therapy

Before going any further, it is important to note that the concept of therapeutic aesthetics as I explore it here is not art therapy and does not address the discipline of art therapy.[7] Art therapy usually involves the analysis of participants' art production in terms of how it might be a portal to the expression of repressed traumas or difficult ideas and how drawing out – in both senses of the word – these traumas enables participants to move forward in their lives. This idea of art therapy is linked to the public reception of certain artists, who are deemed to be, and esteemed for, acting out their traumas and using their art as a means of publicly working through them. In the field of contemporary art, one might think of Tracey Emin, Louise Bourgeois and Yayoi Kusama who all admit to using their work in this way. Interestingly, these are all women artists, though male artists such as Mike Kelley, Robert Gober and Michael Landy could equally be said to publicly work through traumatic experience. However, their 'acting out' is classed as social critique, whereas the aforementioned female artists' works are considered as a direct expression of the personal. This discrepancy highlights the fact that the therapeutic, while popular with audiences, is frowned upon in serious art discourse. From the perspective of the latter, the therapeutic is a feminized and uncritical mode of accounting for personal experience in narratives that structurally oscillate between damage and redemption. For example, in the 1990s, US art historian and critic Hal Foster criticized contemporary art that he considered aped the psychologistic compulsion of therapy culture to speak one's trauma on talk shows and in memoirs (Foster, 1996a: 123–4). His view was that rather than succumbing to the presence-to-self exhorted by such media forms, art's purview revolves around the unrepresentability of trauma, an aesthetic mode that questions conflating identity and/as traumatic experience. And while my goal in this book is not simply to recuperate the therapeutic as an aesthetic mode of criticality, key to my argument is that the performative strategies used in my artists' moving image case studies question the mythemes of aspirational selfhood promulgated in neoliberal cognitive capitalism.

Cognitive capitalism

The term 'cognitive capitalism' is defined by French economist Yann Moulier Boutang as a third form of capitalism – the first two being the mercantile and the industrial – which is founded on 'the accumulation of immaterial capital, the dissemination of knowledge and the driving role of the knowledge economy' (2011: 50). Cognitive capitalism is 'part of a range of new terms which have also tried to question the uncritical identification of the economy with the capitalist economy *tout court* (such as communicative capitalism, semioinfocapitalism, biocapitalism, neoliberal capitalism and such likes)' (Terranova in Neidich, 2013: 47).[8] Terranova takes issue with the term 'cognitive' for not emphasizing the centrality of the affective and the pre-cognitive to the operations of contemporary capitalism and its extraction of surplus value from these immaterial phenomena. However, for me, this is implied by the term given the insistence in contemporary neuroscientific accounts of cognition on automatic and unconscious processing.[9] It could be said that all the terms Terranova lists are united in being various attempts to describe a contemporary capitalist paradigm in which surplus value is extracted from intellectual, immaterial and relational forms of living labour rather than simply from mechanized industrial production. Part of this expansion of the areas of life available for the extraction of surplus value extends to the aesthetic freedom that characterized art as a realm separate from labour in modernist discourse. However, this has not been the case for quite some time.

As Hal Foster put it in 1983, the notion of a general aesthetic realm as a realm separated from the world that acted as 'a critique of the world as it is' (xv) has itself become absorbed and instrumentalized by that very world in which global wars and exploitative conditions are exacerbated. Foster posed the term 'anti-aesthetic' to posit the necessity for a strategy of interference and practice of resistance in the face of such a world (1983: xvi). And rather than this being a definitive position, Foster's proposition of the anti-aesthetic 'signals a practice, cross-disciplinary in nature, that is sensitive to cultural forms engaged in a politic (e.g. feminist art) or rooted in a vernacular – that is, to forms that deny the idea of a privileged aesthetic realm' (Foster, 1983: xv). Such a privileged aesthetic realm is further dismantled by the proximity of contemporary forms of art production, its affective and intellectual labour, to other forms of knowledge production such as 'the global mass of living labor-including activities performed in leisure time such as posting comments, photographs and videos to social networking platforms' (Terranova, 2013: 49). The aesthetics of cognitive capitalism could be said to paradoxically achieve the avant-garde desire to unite art and life, but rather than this being a liberation from labour, it entails an increased subjugation to it. As Terranova goes on to describe:

> From advertising and marketing to the biotech and pharmaceutical industries, from media production to the arts, from care of the body and the self (care of children, the elderly, the sick, beauty and fitness) to the aesthetic production of everyday life (everything pertaining to the home, fashion and style), ultimately, contemporary capitalism implies a real subsumption of the whole of life stretching from the biological life of the species to the spiritual life of publics, from bios to noos, from organic to inorganic life. (2013: 50)

If one accepts this categorization of contemporary life under capitalism, it is not a great stretch of the imagination to consider the numerous psychopathologies incessantly discussed in contemporary media as being connected to this subsumption. I shall have cause to repeat them many times in this book, but Terranova lists them as follows: 'Attention deficit disorder, depression, anxiety, panic, burn-out syndrome, and even new quasi-pathologies such as Internet addiction expose a kind of excess of the life of the psyche with relation to the imperatives of productivity' (2013: 51). Terranova's list tallies with those of other theorists and philosophers whose work will be drawn on in future chapters – Bernard Stiegler, Franco 'Bifo' Berardi, Félix Guattari, Steven Shaviro and Jonathan Beller, amongst others. While this is a list of male heavyweights, I would insist from the outset that my approach is feminist in that I use a questioning method that does not fully subscribe to their use of '"bulldozer" concepts' (Illouz, 2008: 4) such as neoliberal capitalism, biopolitics and semiocapitalism. Although I shall continuously revert to the term cognitive capitalism, I intend it to function as a shorthand reference to a capitalist context that is characterized by the extraction of surplus value from psychological life and in which art functions as another form of immaterial labour, both conditions generating psychopathological symptoms that provide rich material for artists' moving image works.

In conjunction with particular case studies that have informed my thinking of therapeutic aesthetics as pharmacological and as a micro-resistance within neoliberal cognitive capitalism, the philosophical springboard for my argument is Stiegler's engagement with psychoanalyst D.W. Winnicott in *What Makes Life Worth Living: On Pharmacology* (2013a). While my chapters will move away from Stiegler's critique of what he calls consumerist capitalism to foreground artworks as themselves theoretical objects and to focus more on an expanded sense of Winnicott's concept of transitional space, I begin by adopting Stiegler's pharmacological critique whereby he updates Jacques Derrida's discussion of the pharmakon in 'Plato's Pharmacy' (1981).[10]

The pharmakon

The etymology of the Greek word 'pharmakon' as simultaneously referring to both remedy and poison may be familiar to Western academic audiences through its resuscitation in Derrida's essay. In 'Plato's Pharmacy', Derrida engages with the *Phaedrus* in which Plato considers the technology of writing as a poison that contaminates the self-presence or authenticity of speech as the truth of inner experience. In Derrida's deconstructionist reading of *Phaedrus*, he shows, however, that speech is always dependent on an (technological) exteriority that informs the experience of the inside. The outside and the inside are always in a dynamic, enfolding relation to one another rather than a hierarchical or separable one. Writing is both the remedy to memory and the poisoning of memory, its pharmacology being 'the passage among opposing values' (Derrida, 1981: 98). Derrida refers to Thamus in the *Phaedrus* pointing out that 'the *pharmakon* of writing is good for *hypomnesis* (re-memoration, recollection, consignation) and not for the *mneme* (living, knowing memory)' (91). While this condemns it as of little worth in Thamus' eyes, Derrida shows that the medicinal cure of speaking is itself a treatment 'based on recipes learned by heart' (72). And, not only that, but the art of speaking was considered an even better pharmakon than writing by the rhetoricians who used it to sway audiences rather than to testify to the truth of inner experience. As Elizabeth Wilson in her critique of antidepressants writes: 'Derrida's analysis of the pharmakon brings our attention to how this word always signifies in more than one direction: it can never mean just "remedy" without also meaning "poison" and "philter". [...] it is not possible to ... heal' (2015: 143). Although I shall not be looking at pharmaceuticals per se, Wilson's conclusion that antidepressants are 'one mode of remedy-poison in a system of depressing differences, alliances, partialities, and disjunctions' (145–6) echoes my counterintuitive notion that the therapeutic aesthetics enacted in and by my artists' moving image case studies are conflictual and ambivalent, both toxic and curative in one and the same measure.[11] To develop my argument, I append the concept of performativity, which I would say is inherently pharmacological, to therapeutic aesthetics.

Performativity

The concept of performativity is best known in Western academic circles in its derivation from feminist philosopher Judith Butler's 1990s reworking of linguist J.L. Austin's speech acts in conjunction with Derrida's insistence on the instability of the sign.[12] Although Austin would later say that all speech acts are performative to one degree or another, the generally held view of performativity is based on his initial categorization of speech into constative and performative acts, the former tending to describe and make statements that can be validated as being true or false, while the latter to enact a situation, thereby instituting a change of state in a ritualistic, social and/or legal context. For example, the speech act 'I sentence you to three years in prison' executes its action at the same time as the utterance. The impetus of Butler's reformulation of Austin's performative speech acts was to suggest that identity norms are consolidated by the repetitive iteration of learned behaviours and rituals. Rather than being essential to the subject, identity is 'performatively constituted by the very expressions that are said to be its results' (Butler, 1990: 25). Thereby, performativity exposes 'the instability and incompleteness of subject-formation' (Butler, 1993: 226).

The version of performativity I shall deploy in this book refers to both Butler's emphasis on language and its more commonsensical meaning as theatrical performance. In this, I follow Eve Kosofsky Sedgwick. While acknowledging Butler's distinction between performativity and performance, i.e. that in performativity there is no doer behind the deed, Sedgwick writes that the 'line between words and things or between linguistic and nonlinguistic phenomena is endlessly changing, permeable and entirely unsusceptible to any definitive articulation' (2003: 6). The mutability of performativity in both linguistic and theatrical performances prevents identity from being reified as an object and applied to subjects in the discourses of health and well-being that predominate as techniques of governance in cognitive capitalism. My further attraction to the term is that my case studies, whether they be documentary or narrative or a mix of the two, all encompass speech acts: linguistic and/or gestural; scripted and/or improvised.

While performativity destabilizes the notion of an authentic subject, on the other hand, it 'has to do with repetition, very often the repetition of oppressive and painful gender norms ....This is not freedom, but a question of how to work the trap that one is inevitably in' (Butler in Liz Kotz 1992: 84). This may not sound very hopeful, but as Nikolas Rose, a sociologist who reads Butler very closely, asserts: 'capacities for action emerge out of the specific regimes and technologies that machinate humans in diverse ways' (1998: 185). Rather than seeing these regimes and technologies as immutable, he claims that they 'can produce all the effects of resistance, appropriation, utilization, transformation, and transgression' (Rose, 1998: 185), but these cannot be predicted or known in advance of their action. As Butler says: 'there is no easy way to know whether something is subversive [...] for a copy to be subversive of heterosexual hegemony it has to both mime and displace its conventions' (in Kotz, 1992: 84). Performativity then is inherently pharmacological in the sense that any displacement of conventions that might occur in the act of mimicry is also in part a reiteration of them.

Homeopathic mimicry

Questions of gender do not predominate in my book, but mimicry does, a subtext of my argument being that in order to transform the poisons that circulate in cognitive capitalism, therapeutic aesthetics involves the treatment of like with like. In other words, artworks mime the psychopathological excesses of the system to both critique and displace its advocacy of positivity and denial of deleterious effects. Here, I appropriate Steven Shaviro's term 'homeopathic magic' to discuss artists' moving image works in terms of the creation of worlds that mimetically exacerbate the psychopathologies endemic to cognitive capitalism and, in the process of performing survivance, proffer a conflictual remedy to them. But, as Lauren Berlant puts it in relation to her studies of literary fiction:

> The key here is not to see what happens to aesthetically mediated characters as equivalent to what happens to people but to see that in the affective scenarios of these works and discourses we can discern claims about the situation of contemporary life. (Berlant, 2011: 9)

Methodology and chapter outline

The 'therapeutic turn' (Madsen, 2014) that originates in cultural and social discourse in the United States and the United Kingdom in the 1960s and 1970s, in which an ethos of self-actualization replaces transcendent (collective) structures of meaning, partly occurs as a result of the dispersal of psychology and psychoanalysis into countercultural ideas of liberated selfhood. However, other than some discussion of Winnicott's ideas and reference to the work of psychiatrist Félix Guattari, I will not be using a psychoanalytic methodology, my focus being on how media practices disseminate the 'talking cure' as speech acts and gestures performed in the public spaces of the gallery or online. I take as read that the 'talking cure' has become a public form of popular discourse in both political life and cultural representation from reality TV to artists' moving image. In each chapter, I stage an encounter or encounters between theoretical concepts and moving image artworks that perform a pharmacological oscillation between therapeutics as an adaptive mimicry of dominant ideology and therapeutics as potential transformation. Chapter 2 will expand on Stiegler's analysis of the pharmakon in relation to Winnicott's transitional object, but, more importantly, given the dependence of my argument on moving image art encounters, it will perform one such encounter with a video installation by Pipilotti Rist. This short chapter acts as both a supplement to this introduction and a preamble to the pharmacological aesthetics that will be homeopathically administered in the following eight chapters.

Chapter 3 will feature two works by artist and filmmaker Harun Farocki. Exploring the imbrication of poison and cure in the techniques and technologies of what Farocki refers to as 'commodity capitalism', I shall argue that Farocki's therapeutic aesthetics is to present technical images as homeopathic doubles of contemporary conditions that 'look at which things are happening and under which contradictions' (Farocki in Eshun, 2012: 78). The pharmacological aspect of this non-judgmental looking becomes especially poignant in relation to Farocki's gallery installation *Serious Games* in which industrial pharmaka are used to both train for war and develop a cure for one of its aftermaths, PTSD. In Chapter 4, I continue to develop the pharmacological aesthetics of war-themed moving image in relation to Omer Fast's gallery film installations *The Casting* and *5000 Feet is the Best*, both of whose narratives revolve around PTSD symptomatology. Inspired by interviews with real soldiers and a drone operator respectively, Fast's invented narrations mimic and disperse the symptoms of trauma – flashbacks and dissociative projections – across the transitional space of the works. I argue that in inventing narratives that creatively mimic its symptoms, Fast's work provides an inoculation of trauma that enables viewers to immerse themselves in a space that they would otherwise distance themselves from.[13] To develop this idea further, I contrast Fast's work to the overtly therapeutic ethos of Kryzstof Wodiczko's *Abraham Lincoln: War Veteran Projection, Union Square* (2012), which seeks to raise consciousness about the traumatic effects of war on the psyche in the hope of preventing it.

Homeopathic mimicry is furthered explored in Chapter 5 in relation to Melanie Gilligan's online and gallery serial video works in which she allegorizes life under cognitive capitalism. Deploying a kind of sci-fi realism to narrate the damaging psychic effects of immaterial labour and its attendant technologies on the human sensorium, Gilligan's allegories speculatively map the 'invisible abstractions' (Shaviro, 2010: 6) that drive the globalized economy.[14] Mapping this vertiginous terrain is somewhat remedial in itself, but Gilligan's therapeutic aesthetics offers more than a diagnosis. Immersing themselves in the flows and chains of speculative capital, her characters probe the possibilities of existing, not outside of it, but beyond it. Gilligan's pharmacological aesthetics imagines a collective subjectivity as both solution and problem, cure and poison. Added to this, the experimental nature of her post-cinematic aesthetic which incorporates television, cinema and the internet, when viewed through the lens of Guattari's notion of 'mixed semiotics', suggests how her work might be read as resisting, while mimicking, dominant forms of signification in cognitive capitalism.

In Chapter 6, I address the therapeutic emotional style that operates in political and media public discourse. Liz Magic Laser's theatrical remediations of televised political rhetoric by journalists and politicians expose how scripted performances deploying such a style are used to manipulate and control channels of power. I explore whether her aesthetic of homeopathic mimicry represents our powerlessness in relation to political rhetoric, but in a way that allows us to masochistically enjoy it, or whether it has a more pharmacological dimension. In my encounter with her film installation *Primal Speech*, I put Franco 'Bifo' Berardi's notion of exhausted withdrawal from the sphere of production into dialogue with Winnicott's notion of the transitional object as transformative. Laser's use of the psy therapy of life coaching in the film in conjunction with material objects in the installation is, I argue, suggestive of an imaginative projection beyond the frame of unconscious identifications with political leaders based on parental imagos. From this chapter on, there is a shift in my oscillation between the remedial and poisonous poles of the pharmakon towards an emphasis on the former. While small homeopathic doses of a more remedial nature are drip-fed throughout the book, chapters up to this point weigh more heavily on diagnosis and critique, a pharmacological approach encapsulated by Stiegler's response to seeing Alain Resnais' *Same Old Song* (1997). For him, the final moments of the film 'when the characters articulate [...] the sickness from which they suffer are for us a moment of well-being. Phew! It's said. It's out. Our illness has been articulated' (2014: 41). In giving the silent suffering of isolated individuals a social context, the external filmic projection of the sickness inherent in the socio-economic order provides some solace.

Interestingly, my shift in emphasis obliquely relates to the fact the artists' moving image case studies that I explore in the final four chapters stage encounters between 'real' participants rather than actors. These 'real' situations are not modes of socially engaged practice or the recuperation of 'the nicer procedures of our service economy' (Foster, 2004: 21–2) in relational aesthetics, but are filmic performances of group psychic space. Chapter 7 focuses on Leigh Ledare's documentary film projects *The Large Group (Zurich)* and *The Task*, in which he sets up encounter groups based on the Tavistock Institute's principles as initially set down by psychoanalyst Wilfred Bion. These films could be said to perform an alternative kind of collective subjectivity to the fictional ones explored in Gilligan's work. Facilitating the acting out of projections and prejudices within these artificial group settings, Ledare's films operate like public clinics that invite viewers to vicariously participate in the dynamics of control and problem-solving that coheres on-screen. Referring to Guattari's theories of group dynamics, which align somewhat with Bion's, I argue that Ledare's films are artistic models of how a group might constitute itself as a transitional space. Although Guattari spoke negatively about audio-visual media environments, he nonetheless posited their potential in performing deindividuated speech acts whereby the subject becomes 'a collective agent of utterance' (Guattari, 2015: 70) rather than being the sole possessor of a personological symptomatology.[15]

Well-being is both an aspirational value and a desirable commodity, the lack of which marks a subject out as failing to live according to the ideals of 'achievement society'. Chapters 8 and 9 focus more on the curative side of the pharmacological without foregoing the inherent toxicity that cognitive capitalism attempts to shore up by the catch-all term 'well-being'. Chapter 8 centres on two artists who use others in their work: one as a stand-in for the self – Gillian Wearing's experimental documentary *Self Made*; the other, Oriana Fox's *The O Show*, which features the artist as a chat show host with invited guests. In Wearing's film, method acting is used as a potential tool of liberation for seven participants who re-enact painful memories in the workshops led by method acting coach Sam Rumbelow. Rather than viewing these re-enactments as a cathartic purgation of negative emotions that would enable a subject to live well according to neoliberal norms, I argue that the film's therapeutic aesthetics lies in its exploration of creative fabulation, i.e. the capacity to performatively play with one's 'truth'. Fox's use and advocacy of REBT on *The O Show*, which is filmed live with a public audience, while the edited videos are uploaded online, links the therapy's tool of shame-attacking to artistic methods of 'exposure therapy' as a way of overcoming problems. Rather than this being an adaptation to the injunction in cognitive capitalism to be successful, I argue that Fox, and the artists I focus on in Chapters 9 and 10, Lucy Beech and Rehana Zaman, enact feminist homeopathic treatments to alleviate, but not eradicate, the ills of subjects who are doubly trapped under the dictates of neoliberal capital.

Feminized bodies are deployed in neoliberal capitalist logic to represent the desire for and the necessity of constant self-improvement, but they are also the bodies called upon to perform immaterial labour as an unpaid or underpaid form of therapeutic emotional style within neoliberal institutions and corporations. Chapter 9 explores the pharmacological tension that exists between the desire to succeed and its toxic stakes in a number of works by Beech, concluding with a discussion of the transitional pleasures that might be involved in immaterial labour despite its commodification of affective experiences. I argue that while neoliberal capital blurs the boundaries between the productive and the reproductive, it does not commodify everything. In the same chapter, Zaman's videos suggest how performative modes of recognition and misrecognition might create transitional pockets of well-being that enable survivance[16] despite subjection to the toxicities of discrimination on the basis of race, class or gender. Rather than aligning these pockets of well-being to the current ubiquity of self-care in art and critical discourse, in my final chapter I situate them in relation to what cultural critic Lauren Berlant calls 'the mode of enacting life through habituated gestures that stretch the present out so that enjoyment is possible, a kind of autopoetic, proprioceptive dressage' (2011: 63). Berlant's inference here relates to acts of poetic autonomy that take place within the compromised spaces of everyday existence; however, I would maintain that the performative play enabled by artists' moving image works also transforms the everyday, not as a transcendental aesthetic, but by creating a space in which identitarian categories that damage and harm can be shifted slightly. For me, this trajectory links to the ambivalent aesthetics of healing that Susan Buck-Morss describes as not meaning 'whole. It just means capable of responding to the present possibilities for happiness' (in Buck-Morss and Kester, 1997: 45). She is not referring to art; in fact, she describes the liquidation of art in technologies of reproduction, but to aesthetic practices, what she calls a philosophical anthropology of the everyday (43). While the works I look at are mainly shown in art galleries and sometimes online, I suggest that their performative therapeutic modalities, in miming subjection to cognitive capitalism's socio-economic order, paradoxically alleviate its psychopathologies, albeit transitionally. This process has to be distinguished from art therapy as an instrument of use in which individuals may, as

Guattari asserts, be encouraged to reconcile themselves to their 'biological contingencies' and integrate 'into the status quo' (2015 [1972]: 82).

Therapeutic aesthetics as a performative modality suspends the goal of a cure. Utilizing the same capitalist imaginary and its stereotypes and clichés, the moving image artworks in this book repurpose them. Therapeutic aesthetics has to do with how the fictional enactment of therapeutic techniques and forms in moving image artworks might allow both on- and off-screen participants to gain a perspective on and reimagine the traumas of emotional life under cognitive capitalism. Its affirmative nature has to do with the exhibition of survival in the face of a techno-political governance that engenders the very anxieties, depressions and post-traumatic stress disorders that it aims to eradicate by means of state-sanctioned cognitive behavioural therapies. While such healing is necessary, the values of rampant individualism, competition and acquisition of social capital that underpin this rationale also need to be kept in the frame so that, as Elizabeth Wilson puts it, the 'harm that is always at the scene of remedial action' (2015: 144) is acknowledged. In this way, resistance is kept alive without destroying the remedial pleasures of the pharmakon.

2

Setting the scene – two supplementary vignettes

Worry will vanish

Before going on to my main case studies, I want to describe an encounter with Pipilotti Rist's *Worry Will Vanish Horizon* (2014) that was instrumental to my thinking. As a supplementary vignette, this encounter allows me to introduce my methodological approach as one that departs from what Sedgwick calls 'the hermeneutics of suspicion' (2003: 140) and invests in what Illouz refers to as 'immanent critique' (20).[1] In contemporary artists' moving image work, the hermeneutics of suspicion would be to enact a Brechtian-like exposé of the image as a mediated form of representation and to take a self-reflexive distanciation from it. As opposed to this, immanent critique explores relations between things from within the context in which they are embedded whether this be within the image apparatus or within a 'real-life encounter'. As Illouz puts it: 'Immanent critique must emerge from a "thick" understanding of people's desires and goals and cannot bracket the actual understandings and strategies of lay actors' (2008: 20). In immanent critique, the artist's desires, and by proxy the audiences, are embedded within and generated in relation to the image apparatus. For me, Rist's videos bypass 'a hermeneutics of suspicion' to proffer regenerative imaginary bodies in immersive audio-visual environments which are both emancipatory and repressive in relation to the codification of identity in neoliberal capitalism. Given her previous punkish mimicry of representations of female stereotypes in order to remedy their toxicity, it was no surprise that she would be attracted to a more overtly therapeutic aesthetic ethos.

For this installation, Rist drew on

> principles of Autogenic training to facilitate a process of relaxation, a technique developed in 1932 by the German psychiatrist Johannes Heinrich Schultz. Autogenic Training involves a repeated set of visualizations, practiced in recommended postures (including lying down), which are intended to alleviate stress.[2]

Projected full-scale on two adjacent gallery walls in front of which a number of beans bags were strewn, the video's imagery featured an acidic hued jungle or garden through which body-parts of a monstrous humanoid, exo-skeletal form occasionally appeared. The rhythm of the editing, its flowing movement of coloured pixels of flora and fauna, moved to the beat of a meditative soundtrack, the atmosphere being akin to a club chill-out room, as viewers, including me, lay on the bean bags transfixed.[3]

I had mentioned to a fellow university lecturer that I was going to see Rist's solo exhibition 'Worry Will Vanish' at Hauser and Wirth, London, in 2015 after a stressful day at work. 'But isn't her work just eye candy for the masses?' he responded, 'Isn't it just pure spectacle without any politics?' I refer to his response here as it unwittingly repeats Marxist theorist Jonathan Beller's critique of the female character's relation to video technology in Wim Wenders' film *Until the End of the World* (1991). All consider immersive video as creating spectacles that channel, or as Stiegler might say, canalize, desire

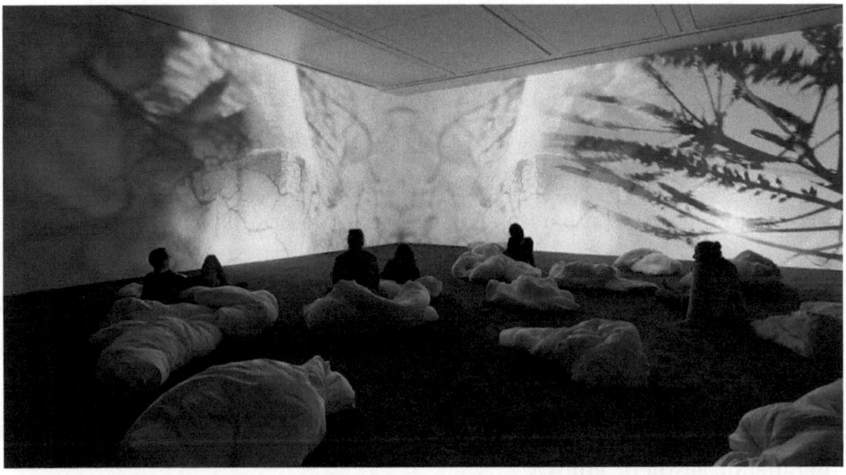

Figure 2.1 Pipilotti Rist, *Worry Will Vanish*, 2014. © Pipilotti Rist. Courtesy the artist, Hauser & Wirth and Luhring Augustine.

into prevailing conditions of consumption. Beller maintains that Wenders uses his female protagonist's empathetic connection to video technology to critique the passive consumption of spectacle as a form that obscures real life and action.[4] Interestingly, the screenplay was co-written by Wenders and Solveig Donmartin, who plays the female protagonist, Claire Tourneur, a researcher developing video technology to enable the blind to see. Video, as evidenced by footage in the film shot with a Sony camcorder, feeds directly into Claire's dream world and according to Beller she develops:

> an addiction to the ghostly, colored electronic shadows of her own pixilated dreams that flicker on her eye-screen [...] Endlessly she watches the movement of the abstracted forms of her desire mediated and motivated only by technology and her own *narcissism* rather than seeking an encounter with the outer world through another visual subject. (2006: 218, emphasis in original)

For Beller, Claire is immersed in the spectacle of her own unconscious, a hallucinogenic temporality characterized by incessant fluidity and plasticity. He claims that her desire is 'pre-symbolic and in certain respects a result of capital's penetration of the infantile' (218).

Worry Will Vanish Horizon could be said to present such an infantile vision in its use of projections in which body parts and flora float and sway dreamily to a hypnotic beat without any fissure of self-reflexivity at the level of the medium that might induce critical consciousness in the spectator. The restful effects of Rist's luscious space could be said to be similar to those experienced in a yoga or mediation class, both activities that are recommended and often organized in the contemporary workplace as offering respite from its environmental conditions of stress. However, unlike the kinds of stress relievers such as yoga and mindfulness advocated by and available in many metropolitan workplaces, in the installation, I was relieved of the responsibility to be a good meditator or yoga practitioner, that is, to make these activities productive in redressing work overload. The relaxation induced by *Worry Will Vanish Horizon* was more akin to how dreams, while being useful in enabling sleep, also open us up to bio-rhythms that are non-productive, i.e. useless from the point of view of extracting economic value from emotional life. Rist's reorientation of somatic and psychic energy, while somewhat in allegiance with managerial injunctions to remedy the exploitative excesses of precarious labour, nonetheless had a side effect that was not reducible to this logic. It allowed for a withdrawal of one's labour and a contingent absorption in a waking dream life with others. This more pharmacological dimension of the video paradoxically tallies with an underexplored aspect of Beller's analysis of Wenders' film.

As Beller himself admits, *Until the End of the World* does not adequately explore the possible potential of Claire's unavailability to heterosexist patriarchy in her immersion in the 'flattening out of the space between the unconscious and representation' (2006: 219). To attend to this potential would be to bypass the binary choice Beller sets up between a 'techno-feminist narcissism blind to issues of political economy, or sexist Marxism constitutionally opposed to experience beyond the purview of the phallic subject' (222). Repurposing this 'choice' in relation to Rist's *Worry Will Vanish Horizon*, I suggest that the generation of an experience 'beyond the purview of the phallic subject' in her work has an inherently therapeutic value for subjects who are considered or consider themselves minoritarian in relation to the dominant order of patriarchal capitalism. As opposed to Beller for whom in relation to visual culture, '[t]herapy is a lost cause – our ironic detachment from belief in reality is already the "cure"' (165), I would want to maintain that the un-ironic absorption in Rist's visual cornucopia has another kind of therapeutic value in facilitating willing spectators to momentarily withdraw from the strictures and speeds of capital in a collective uncodified dreamspace. (Of course, economic consumption also operates in this space, but that is not the target of my pharmacological approach.) Rather than seeing *Worry Will Vanish Horizon* as providing relaxation so that I can go back to work refreshed, the work could equally be said to allow for a reclaiming of bodily energies denied in the life world of neoliberal cognitive capitalism in which such energy is subjected to measurement and control. Aware that 'pure subversion is no longer possible because our reality is too complex and separate: it is already subversive in itself' (Rist in Jones, 2006: 207), Rist's morphological refraction of the body through digital technology can be seen as a form of therapeutic resistance in a culture which is based on the denial of female bio-rhythms and temporalities. Her pixelated body composites are oneiric and joyously regressive. While I do not discuss Rist's work in future chapters, I will return at the end of this book to the idea of therapeutic aesthetics as a form of rhythmanalysis that performs a micro-resistance to the time of quantification.[5] My argument is that moving image artworks that import therapeutic discourses proffer such transformatively conflictual spaces.

What makes life worth living

Although he does not discuss contemporary art, the springboard for my argument is Bernard Stiegler's appropriation of Winnicott's concept of transitional phenomenon in *What Makes Life Worth Living: On Pharmacology*. This appropriation leads Stiegler to move from the kind of Marxist-informed suspicion of audio-visual technology that characterizes Beller's analysis of Wenders' film. On the one hand, Stiegler situates the culture industries in capitalism as perpetuating social and psychic alienation (2013a: 15). In this, he repeats earlier historical Marxist analyses such as those by The Frankfurt School which maintained that 'mass media and television work as pacifying communicators of dominant ideology' (Yates in Bainbridge et al., 2014: 10). However, unlike, for example, Adorno and Horkheimer, Stiegler also maintains that it is 'regressive' to think of any of the culture industries phenomena as a poison destroying interior experience as 'interiority is constituted through the internalisation of a transitional exteriority that precedes it' (2013a: 20). Stiegler refers to this exteriority as technics which are the technologies that allow for the transmission of experience across generations, whether one is referring to manual tools or audio-visual environments. For Stiegler, the human is dependent on these prosthetic means of transmission, the issue being that in our hyperindustrial societies, technics is thoroughly industrialized in the context of an increasingly totalitarian capitalism. However, Stiegler is also critical of Adorno and Horkheimer, positing that they 'ignore the pharmacological character of technics in general and the psycho-technics implemented by the culture industry in particular' (2013a: 15). Psycho-technics, rather than simply destroying interior experience, facilitate it and not necessarily in the direction of consumer capitalism. For Stiegler, a pharmacological approach to culture entails thinking of the pharmakon as a substance that acts as both a poison and a medicine. Elaborating Derrida's reading of the pharmakon in relation to technology, Stiegler argues that the 'hypomnesic', i.e. the technologies of recording memory, is that which constitutes the condition of the 'anamnesic', i.e. remembrance or reminiscence (Stiegler, 2013a: 19). For him, the remedial side of the pharmakon's opposing poles entails returning a sense of control to people's knowledge of how to live, which he claims has been destroyed, i.e. poisoned, by the marketization of life. Stiegler combines his deconstructive philosophical take on the pharmakon with Winnicott's concept of transitional phenomenon to explore the therapeutics of technics (mnemonic technologies) that are needed in a society that Stiegler sees as sick and in need of care.

Stiegler adopts Winnicott's transitional object as itself a kind of mnemonic technology that supports individuation. Winnicott, in his infamous essay *Transitional Objects and Transitional Phenomena: A Study of the First Not-Me Possession* (1953), discusses the infant's process of individuation by means of a transitional object that enables him/her to shift from inner fantasy to outer reality. This process occurs in the intermediate area of experiencing called transitional space. This zone of experience is neither inside nor outside but is, for Winnicott, a process of reality-making that is intrinsically creative, related as it is to the infant's sense of play. The whole process, while in one sense being separate from the mother, is nonetheless facilitated by what Winnicott variably calls the mother-environment or the good-enough mother. In Stiegler's appropriation of Winnicott, the mother-environment becomes a media-environment, thereby colonizing transitional space by the audio-visual objects of the media. This audio-visual environment captures the attention of the human, channelling it into images directed at marketing and consumption. Stiegler calls this psychopower, which he describes as short-circuiting the sublimatory, transindividual processes of creativity and subjecting life to systems of rationalistic management and control (2013a: 32). Rather than the sublimatory, transindividual processes of creativity which enable the transmission of cultural memory beyond the lifespan of the individual, Stiegler claims that the 'premature immersion of the child's psychic apparatus in audiovisual pharmacological milieu short-circuits or bypasses this relation of care […] audiovisual transitional space is purely and simply toxic for the child's brain' (Stiegler, 2013a: 69). Yet, on the other hand, these audio-visual 'pharmaka' are potentially the very objects that might facilitate care by producing intensities 'that traverse and form by opening up [frayant] networks' that are not simply captured by the logic of the market (Stiegler, 2013a: 72).[6] And in fact this is what I claim in relation to my encounter with Rist's *Worry Will Vanish Horizon*, i.e. that the immersive installation did indeed produce such non-productive intensities or oneiric bio-rhythms that are more on the side of individuation than co-option to market values. Although I shall have occasion in future chapters to critique the unwritten gender bias underlying Stiegler's adoption of Winnicott, here I just want to note that he follows Winnicott in placing the responsibility of care in relation to transitional space on the mother, accusing capitalism of transforming the 'sexed body into becoming pure labour force' (2013a: 127). In this, Stiegler rather conservatively implies that the phenomenon of working mothers might deprive the infant of the maternal nurturance of transitional space that mitigates the toxic effects of the object as pharmakon.

However, Winnicott's transitional object is never simply a benign teddy-bear or blanket but is in part a fantastical object that facilitates the enactment and projection of infantile aggression or aggressivity. Referring to Winnicott's idea that transitional space is a site of conflict, Stiegler says that '[t]he *pharmakon* is at once what *enables* care to be taken and that *of which* care must be taken [...] its power is *curative to the immeasurable extent* [...] that is it also destructive' (2013a: 4, original emphasis). However, Stiegler rather problematically, albeit correctly, argues that Winnicott

> showed that the transitional object, which is the condition of the formation of the infantile psychic apparatus, can also become a *pathogenic* factor if the mother fails to locate the therapeutic value of the object, thereby allowing it to become an object of pure addiction. (2013b, online)

Stiegler also insists that it is not a case of returning to a more natural 'maternal-environment', but of developing what he calls a new organology of the senses that would not be propped on the consumptive-appetite drive of psychopower. This new organology of the senses relates specifically to Stiegler's notion of aesthetics.

Stiegler's aesthetics

In 'The Forgetting of Aesthetics: Individuation, Technology, and Aesthetics in the Work of Bernard Stiegler', Bram Leven articulates the shift in Stiegler's thinking from an emphasis on memory to an emphasis on aesthetics. Although Stiegler does not explicitly refer to aesthetics in *What Makes Life Worth Living*, Leven's summary of Stiegler's aesthetics in *Technics and Time 2: Disorientation* (2009) echoes Stiegler's pharmacological approach to technics in the former book. Rather than Kant's transcendental aesthetics which depend on *a priori* concepts of space and time, Stiegler 'accords a central place to technology within the organisation of space and time [that] presupposes an aesthetic ground for individuation' (Leven, 2012: 80). Stiegler's conception of aesthetics bypasses a theory of the beautiful, instead proffering aesthetics as an interplay of rhythms that are lived and experienced via technological mediation. As Leven says:

> There is a sensuous or physiological part, a technical or technological part, and a symbolic or figurative part. The interplay between these three should be seen as an interlacing of different rhythms: biological or physiological rhythms, the manipulation of those rhythms with technology, and finally cultural rhythms that are based both on the biological and technological conditions. (2012: 76–7)

In light of this, it is interesting to note that the etymology of the term 'aesthetics' derives from a combination of 'Aisthitikos', the ancient Greek word for 'perceptive by feeling' and 'aisthisis', the sensory experience of perception (Buck-Morss, 1992: 6).[7] Tracing its genealogy in the eighteenth-century aesthetic theories of Alexander Baumgarten, who, prior to Kant, first developed the aesthetic as a thematic in philosophy, Buck-Morss argues that the original field of the latter was the corporeal and material nature of the life world and the human sensorium. As I have said, for Stiegler, this field is thoroughly technologized, as it was for Walter Benjamin, the subject of Buck-Morss' essay 'Aesthetics and Anaesthetics: Walter Benjamin's Artwork Essay Reconsidered' (1992). Although Stiegler only mentions him in passing, Benjamin's aesthetics could be said to be equally pharmacological and to provide historical precedence for this kind of approach to culture. Not only did Benjamin propose that film technology, in replicating the shocks of modern life, enables us to cope with them by training our perception, he also articulated this 'cure' in terms of narcotic insulation. As Buck-Morss writes: 'technology doubles back on the senses as protection in the form of illusion, taking over the role of the ego in order to provide defensive insulation' (1992: 22). This insulation is necessary for survival in the face of sensory overload in modern life. As well as film, for Benjamin, aesthetic experience in modern life is managed by means of a vase array of anaesthetic technologies consisting of 'drugs and therapeutic practices, from opium, ether, and cocaine to hypnosis, hydrotherapy and electric shock' (Buck-Morss, 1992: 18). These anaesthetics, including film, could be called homeopathic in that they involve administering one kind of poison, i.e. drug, to mitigate another, i.e. the poisonous shocks endemic to what Benjamin refers to as modern experience.

Stiegler also uncannily repeats Benjamin's utopianism in not thinking of the insulating aspects of anaesthetics as a purely negative, narcissistic phenomenon, but as potentially enhancing experience in singular ways, saying that 'before being a pathology, narcissism conditions the *psyche*, desire, and singularity' (Stiegler, 2011a: 59). While capitalism homogenizes desire by canalizing the projections of primordial narcissism, technology can be repurposed to open up the singularity of desire. Stiegler's example of repurposing technology is the creation of open source software; however, he also makes the intriguing suggestion relevant to this book that the poisonous nature of industrial pharmaka might be alleviated in artistic practice that redoubles this poison, claiming that thereby 'a detoxifying suspension may be produced' (2013a: 49).

Not only does this idea of redoubling echo Benjamin's therapeutics of technology, but it also has affinity with Steven Shaviro's notion of homeopathic magic, which will feature alongside Stiegler in the next chapter. Referring to the digital modulations Grace Jones' body undergoes in the video performance of her song 'Corporate Cannibal' (2008), Shaviro claims that 'Jones and [Nick] Hooker perform a feat of homeopathic magic' (2010: 32) that replicates and makes tangible the hyperbolically present, yet virtual abstraction of networks of global capitalism. Shaviro describes the fragmenting and morphing of Jones' body in this video as mimicking the extraction of surplus value from the life world of emotional and reproductive labour. For him, her black and white pixelated mutating body, while being unremittingly subject to the disfiguring modulations of digital technology, nonetheless always bounces back in new iterations that challenge subjection to the apparatus. For Shaviro, such moving image works,[8] in rising to the challenge of immersing themselves in the flows and chains of speculative capital, probe the possibilities of existing beyond it, this aesthetic modality generating a resilient body that he aligns with a hope of resistance. In the following chapters, I adapt the phrase 'homeopathic magic' to discuss how artists' moving image works performatively mimic the conditions of cognitive capitalism not in order to simply reveal them, but to proffer a way of 'using' them for potentially life-enhancing purposes. However, in my pharmacological approach, this has as much to do with the bio-rhythms of the non-productive body that I encountered in Rist's *Worry Will Vanish Horizon* as it has to do with resilience which, when thought of in isolation, becomes another desirable attribute in cognitive capitalism – no matter what harm is enacted on your body, you will always come bouncing back. In the following chapters, withdrawal from normative strictures of productivity will be evidenced through the performativity of speech rather than dream.

3

The imbrication of poison and cure in Harun Farocki

This chapter focuses on the pharmacological aesthetics of poison and cure in relation to two works by artist filmmaker Harun Farocki: the documentary *How to Live in the FRG* (1990) and his gallery installation *Serious Games* (2009–2010). While my main focus is on the latter work, I begin with *How to Live in the FRG* because of its uncanny resonance with Stiegler's assertion that, due to the marketization of life, 'knowledge-how-to-live' is lost in what he refers to as totalitarian capitalism. Farocki's documentary consists of a compilation of fast-paced sequences portraying the kinds of behavioural training necessary to live in what Farocki calls 'the commodity society'. Although there is no voice-over or intertitles, Farocki's montage implies a critical gaze; however, in my reading of the film according to a pharmacological aesthetic, I propose that rather than subjection to the commodity, *How to Live in the FRG* documents a new sense of 'knowledge-how-to-live' as transmitted between institutions and their users. In the second section of this chapter, I explore the pharmacological imbrication of poison and cure in relation to *Serious Games* (2009–2010). The work's presentation of how advanced technology, i.e. virtual imaging, is used to train soldiers for war as well as rehabilitate them in its traumatic aftermath makes it difficult to uphold the dialectical tension between poison and cure, given that, in this context, the necessity of the latter only arises due to and as further preparation for the poison of war. However, even in this case, Farocki's 'immanent' critique of images by means of images, rather than being a transcendental judgment that categorizes poison and cure as oppositional, retains their imbrication. I argue that, rather than moralizing, Farocki's therapeutic aesthetics proffers technical images as homeopathic doubles of contemporary conditions that 'just look at which things are happening and under which contradictions' (Farocki in Eshun, 2012: 78).

How to Live in the FRG

> A man applies for a job. It is not long before he speaks of his having had an alcohol problem some years before, and he declares not only that he no longer drinks, but that he is in therapy and is attending self-help groups. Instead of salary and work experience, the soul is spoken about, because business enterprise affiliates itself to therapeutic enterprise.
>
> (Farocki in Ehmann and Eshun, 2009: 164)

Farocki is here explicitly referring to *How to Live in the FRG*. Although on one level specific to the German society he documents in 1989, the film also more generally records the management of behaviour via the 'therapeutic emotional style' that Illouz identifies as becoming widely available from the mid-twentieth century, not only to individuals, but also to corporations and organizations, as a means of understanding and controlling the self and its interactions with others. The attraction of 'therapeutic language' was its potential to 'organise manager-worker relationships in a nonconfrontational way, and neutralise class struggles by casting them in the benign language of emotion and personality' (Illouz, 2008: 87). Although Illouz is mostly positive about how therapeutic language becomes available to multiple users as ways to enhance their understanding of their lives, her choice of words here betrays its dangers, i.e. to eradicate confrontation and critique. While recourse to 'therapeutic language' ostensibly neutralizes the hierarchies of roles and relations across the employer/employee, trainer/learner divide, this shared use can merely give the appearance of democratic space while hierarchical power relations remain firmly and perhaps more insidiously intact. *How to Live in the FRG* exemplifies this pharmacological conundrum. Focusing on the performative gestures and actions of behavioural training, the film is a dissection of the public spaces of modern life in what was then called West Germany – a country Farocki calls 'a training camp in which techniques for living are practiced by the professionally living' (www.facetsdvd.com). Composed entirely of thirty-two short scenes, the one hour and twenty-three–minute film records instructional and training sessions in various organizations and institutions. An example of observational documentary, it comprises rapidly edited sequences of people performing their professional roles in social-welfare offices, schools, clinics, police stations, public administration offices and Federal Defence training sites. For Farocki, these scenarios are readymade 'psycho-dramas, socio-dramas and other hyphenated-science dramas' (Farocki in Ehmann and Eshun, 2009: 164). Many of the situations he records inadvertently involve a therapeutic dynamic: there are repeated sequences showing midwives training prospective parents to take care of new-born babies; other sequences show child psychologists at work and self-help and drama therapy groups. The film can be considered as a record of the changing conditions of labour in post-industrial society and the incursion of the state and public corporations into areas of life that were previously relegated to the private sphere. In such a society, Farocki states that:

> the plasticity of life and work processes decreases everywhere … the rules by which we are supposed to live are increasingly uncertain, and there are more and more games where life is trained, like a sport … in the commodity society, the instruction manual is the only record of theory. (in Ehmann and Eshun 2009: 165)

On one level, *How to Live in the FRG* is historically specific, its interior architectural settings and clothing adding to this sense; however, watching it in the twenty-first century, the film uncannily echoes many of the sociological accounts and critiques of the therapeutic turn published in the 2000s and after. For example, as Ecclestone and Hayes argue in *The Dangerous Rise of Therapeutic Education* (2009), in capitalist consumer society, education is recast as 'learning', the focus being on knowledge acquisition as an (empowering) object of exchange in the market. Echoing Illouz's sentiments above in regard to labour relations, in their view, recasting education as 'learning' appears to offer 'more *benign* instrumental goals than merely developing "human capital" for the labour market' (2009: 50, my emphasis), thereby making the shift from education to the workplace more palatable. Although they are mainly writing about the UK from the 1990s onwards, their focus on the goals of the therapeutic tendency in education to provide the skills not only to succeed in life but also to cope with the demands of a post-industrial consumer capitalist society in which emotional intelligence is an asset (54) resonates for me with the training sequences in Farocki's film. As well as the aforementioned sequences, others show interview training, soldiers training to fire at tanks, waiting staff training for their roles, police altercation re-enactments, management group training and weightwatcher groups, the film being entirely made up of scenes in which 'life was acted to demonstrate something, to instruct, to practice, to exorcise, to cope with something' (Farocki in Ehmann and Eshun, 2009: 164). Farocki's dispassionate camera does not judge these scenes. His expectation is that his audience might make associations between the sequences – some of which are repeated seemingly at random – and so formulate (a critical) awareness of the instructional nature of real-life. As Roswitha Mueller claims, Farocki's observational camera gives viewers room to 'co-fabulate', his (Brechtian) principle of creating breaks between units of framing allowing viewers to attend to what would normally be glossed over (Mueller, 1989: 89).[1] This is Farocki's form of immanent critique by which viewers are interpellated by the relations between images rather than from 'an external perspective from where … a normative judgement of the relation between images and power' might be gleaned (Celis Bueno, 2016: 8). As Claudio Celis Bueno further characterizes it: 'Farocki's immanent critique of images by means of images is thus not a critique of the deceptive power of images but a critique of their concrete role within a given power relation and a given process of subjectification' (2016: 8).[2] While Celis Bueno's critical framework is different from Illouz's notion of immanent critique that I referred to in my introduction, they are linked in their emphasis of critique emerging from within the material relations between things. However, Illouz's reference to the affordances that cultural and technological techniques enable in addressing people's desires and goals moves more in the pharmacological direction of my reading of *How to Live in the FRG*, which is that the process of subjection to training also enables a productive 'subjectivation' (Lazzarato 2014a: 138), i.e. a means by which people enact their agency.[3]

Reading the film as elucidating the processes of subjectification is convincing. For example, *How to Live in the FRG* opens with a sequence showing a pornographic film on a computer screen, the accompanying clicking sound of an off-screen ticker tape timer equating the production of bodily sensation to economic production. Throughout, the sound of timers such as ticker tape and stopwatches is ubiquitous, signalling that all activities are ultimately bound to this form of quantification and value based on the equation between time and money. However, in many of the following sequences, participants appear to be fully identified with and absorbed in the nondramatic performance of their roles, their exploitative aspects being downplayed by the couching of labour time in terms of the therapeutic. Farocki's description of the striptease scene is telling:

> We filmed a man teaching a woman how to strip effectively, and when she is exhausted, he directs her in an exercise which teaches her how to relax. After the attempted titillation comes the therapy. Perhaps the sexual titillation is already a therapeutic measure. (in Ehmann and Eshun 2009: 164)

The film's montage jarringly moves from the striptease to images of a child psychologist engaging a child in play therapy using a variety of toys manufactured for this purpose. There is no commentary, just a deadpan focus on the repetitious gestures of selecting which shape fits into which hole, the child's 'learning' being predetermined by the preformatted choices, a synonym perhaps of adaptation to societal norms. On the one hand, the viewer becomes acutely aware of how collective rituals are governed, how personal emotions and behaviours are turned into objects to be observed and managed. However, on the other hand, the democratic values and potential life-enhancement involved in the training of parents-to-be and the organization of self-help and drama therapy groups for the rehabilitation of addictive or destructive behaviour also emerge. In charting how intimate and singular practices and knowledges of care have become managed by public institutions, which both homogenizes and democratizes them, the film could be said to echo Stiegler's pharmacological approach to the therapeutic in which one and the same substance acts as a poison 'destroying society and proletarianizing human existence, as well as acting as a medicine, producing social ties and deproletarianizing human existence' (Stiegler in Lemmens, 2011: 35). Note that Stiegler's use of the term 'proletarianization' is not necessarily to do with downward social mobility but more to do with the cultural loss of the knowledge of how to make (savoir-faire) and how to live (savoir-vivre). The result of this loss of know-how is that 'consumers [are] discharged of the burden of responsibility for shaping their own lives' and instead lead 'preformatted lifestyles' based on market models (Stiegler in Lemmens, 34).[4] But is that really the case?

On the one hand, the disciplinary nature of regulating and governing life – what Foucault would call biopower – serves the interests of state and corporate powers in controlling both the physical and psychical bodies of populations as well as making their lives available for profitable ends. On the other hand, Farocki's film also shows how the training of behaviour makes a range of skills available to large groups of people, thereby generating the potential for new autonomous subjectivities. While one reading of Farocki's film might view it as being critical of the (therapeutic) use of training as an acquiescence to biopolitical forms of governance, it also presents a more ambiguous, even conflictual, attitude towards this institutional incursion into the everyday life world and the transmission of skills made available for use through (therapeutic) training. Observing how the 'knowledge-how-to-live' that Stiegler refers to is externalized in rituals that train, educate and support people in their daily lives, the film might also suggest that this *institutional* organization of social behaviours potentially enables subjects to put knowledge into action to achieve singular, rather than preformatted, desires and goals. Of interest here is the distinction in French between the terms 'institution' and 'establishment'. In English, an institution is an establishment, whereas in French, an establishment is referred to as *etablissement*, while *institution* is more dynamically associated with assembling and/or constituting relations (Goffey, 2016). Although Goffey discusses this distinction in relation to the work of French psychiatrist Félix Guattari, who will feature in later chapters, I mention it here as it contributes to my point that the institutional production of subjectivity is not necessarily alienating or destructive of autonomy. As Nikolas Rose remarks the 'question of agency', as it has come to be termed, poses a false problem (1998: 185). Rather, 'capacities for action emerge out of the specific regimes and technologies that machinate humans in diverse ways' (Rose, 1998: 186–7). Agency, rather than being autonomous selfhood, is

> a distributed outcome of particular technologies of subjectification that involve human beings as subjects of a certain type of freedom and supply the norms and techniques by which that freedom is to be recognized, assembled, and played out in specific domains. (Rose, 1998: 187)

A telling scene from *How to Live in the FRG* shows two women directing another older woman for her role as a cleaner in a workplace re-enactment. She is asked to repeat a series of gestures from losing her office keys to picking up a telephone, continuously discussing them with her instructors as she performs them. What emerges from this more extended scene in the film is the woman's enjoyment of practising the instructions. It is as if she *institutes* herself through their repetitious execution, becoming one with her role. In his short essay 'Empathy' (2008), Farocki writes that:

> I was similarly surprised in '68, when shooting a film, to see that neither the amateurs nor the professionals could distinguish between themselves and the text; they internalized it faster than they could memorise it [insisting on] speaking a text as if it had sprung from some remote, inaccessible, inner cleft. (in Ehmann and Guerra, 2016: 105)

He then decided to stop preventing actor's or non-actor's identification with the text and instead to follow them in their actions. This again is an example of 'immanent critique' in which relations emerge from the context in which they are already entangled. As media theorist Tim Markham puts it in a different context, as social actors '[w]e find ourselves acting out all sorts of practices of existing before "we" exist' (Markham, 2019: 467).[5] It is this experientially prereflective, but technically informed, sense of existing that enables the making of an intimate connection with distant others predicated on 'the merely felt experience of the other in everyday life – an experience characterised by distraction, ambivalence and unreflexive sentimentality' (2019: 471). Although at this point in my argument it may seem like a leap to claim that the filmic projection of this space of engagement can act as a kind of transitional object, I nonetheless wish to suggest it here.

Film as transitional space

As I discussed in my introduction and in the last chapter, Stiegler combines his elaboration of the pharmacological therapeutics of technics with Winnicott's theory of the transitional object. For Stiegler, today's societal environment is in need of care, akin to the kind facilitated by Winnicott's maternal-environment in which the infant learns to distinguish between fantasy and reality by means of the intermediate area of experience known as transitional space. In the safety of this space, the infant discovers and makes use of transitional objects that are meaningful only to him- or herself, but which allow for the acting out through play activity that enables the journey from fantasy to reality. While this psychoanalytic narrative of infantile psychic life might seem at a remove to the kinds of scenarios being performed in Farocki's film, it is noteworthy that historically in both the United Kingdom and Germany, as well as in the United States, the proliferation and consolidation of therapeutic discourses derived from a post-war context in which 'concern over adjustment and well-being' (Illouz, 2007: 57) were seen as a political imperative to salvage the psychic damage resulting from post-war demoralization and the economic downturn. Specifically, Winnicott's ideas about the role of the maternal or mother-environment in nurturing the infant's transition from illusion to reality can be aligned with the humanitarian impetus in the UK to heal the nation in the wake of the two world wars.[6] However, this drive towards the health of the nation is not without its ideologically moral implications that are in turn replicated in this psychoanalytic narrative of the infant's move from fantasy to reality. Although the transitional object in itself is neither good nor bad, there are preferable outcomes to what Winnicott calls the infant's disillusionment. His idea is that if the mother-environment is good enough, the infant will make good object choices nurturing creativity and religious feeling rather than toxic object choices such as fetishism and other addictions. However, creativity and religious feeling are not immune from toxicity, religious feeling especially being a prime motivator of harm to others, and the history of art is riddled with tales of the imbrication of creativity and aggressivity.

Societal ideals entail the technical production of what are deemed to be desirable subjects. For example, Foucault would refer to the production of docile subjects in disciplinary societies by means of the establishments of the prison, the factory, the school and the psychoanalyst's couch. In Farocki's film, the situations in which training takes place could equally be said to be producing social remedies against toxicity, e.g. the rechannelling of addictive behaviours using overtly therapeutic modalities such as AA meetings, primal scream workshops and drama therapy, as well as the training involved in learning to care for the yet-to-be-born and the use of play in analysing child psychology. The question that arises from the film is whether these remedies are merely productive of docile (or proletarian) subjects or whether they might be productive in ways that are not necessarily normative. While Winnicott does not refer to the kinds of objects that interest me here, i.e. the industrial image-objects that Stiegler calls pharmaka, Bainbridge, Ward and Yates

(2014) use Winnicott's work to show how televisual objects come to function as transitional objects for people in order to process and cope with various problems and issues in their lives in innovative, self-reliant ways. While theirs is a practical and normative approach, my interest is in how performative rituals documented on film might function (for viewer/s) as transitional spaces that enable the incorporation of both toxicity and cure, thereby acknowledging the life-enhancing as well as the life-destroying aspects of the object, or 'technics'. Needless to say, in both my adaptation and Stiegler's, Winnicott's maternal-environment is superseded by the audio-visual environment.

As I mentioned in my introduction, Stiegler suggests that the poisonous nature of industrial 'pharmaka' (image-objects) can be detoxified in artistic practices in their redoubling of audio-visual environments that might otherwise be purely bound to the logic of consumerism (2013a, 49). What is implied in this passing comment is the notion that artistic practices that mimic mainstream audio-visual environments might suspend their appetitive consumerist drive and offer a more reflective space. This is quite a common idea.[7] It can also be related to Farocki's immanent critique, to cite Celis Bueno again, 'of images by means of images [which] appropriates operational images and displaces them from the sphere of a technical process (inscribed always in an institutional network of power) towards *the sphere of contemplation*' (2016: 17, my emphasis). For Stiegler, this sphere is cinema's cathartic function, which, while overburdened by industrialization, is not ruled out by it. The cinematic image retains the capacity of reintroducing the horizon of what Stiegler calls 'the expected, unexpected' (2014: 88), whose impact would re-singularize the subject. Now while this notion of the 'unexpected' suggests an eruption of sorts,[8] in *How to Live in the FRG* the space of projective reflection is more on a continuum with a non-dramatic form of enacting 'knowledge-how-to-live', regardless of the regulatory conditions of these performances. While these could be seen as limitations imposed by the 'commodity society', this does not rule out entrainment enhancing the lives of their performers, for example, the confidence acquired by both men and women in learning how to hold and bathe an infant. While such a skill might have been thought to be both innate to women and passed on through female genealogy, the 'commodity society' liberates women by denaturalizing this knowledge and transforming it into something that can be learnt to make life better. In this sense then, *How to Live in the FRG* shows the pharmacological nature of training as an aesthetic mode of behaviour that cannot be quantified in terms of good or bad. To conclude the first section of this chapter, Farocki's comment on his observational film *An Image* (1983), which was shot for the television program Projektionen 83, is apropos here:

> The television station that commissioned it assumes in these cases that I'm making a film that is critical of its subject matter, and the owner or manager of the thing that's being filmed assumes that my film is an ad for them. I try to do neither. Nor do I want to do something in between, but beyond both. (Farocki in Pantenburg, 2016: 150)

Serious Games (2009–2010)

As opposed to the images of training for life in *How to Live in the FRG*, Farocki's multi-screen installation *Serious Games* shows the use of images for training US soldiers how to kill, and for the equally instructional rehabilitation purposes of 'curing' one of the poisons generated by the military-industrial-technical complex, PTSD.[9] Although Farocki's concept of the 'commodity society' may seem somewhat quaint in relation to contemporary forms of cognitive capitalism, it is notable that Franco 'Bifo' Berardi uses similar terms when referring to the mobilization to wage war as a further engine of capitalist global accumulation in which 'everyday life is ready to be subjected to the unlimited rule of the commodity' (2011: 36). Farocki's interest, however, is in the image as an instrument of war rather than in war itself as is evident in earlier films such as his trilogy *Eye/Machine* (2001–2003) and *War at a Distance* (2003). In proffering the notion that war is 'produced by workers acting on instruction' (Chinen, 2014), the installation connects across time with the training scenarios documented in *How to Live in the FRG*.

Serious Games consists of four projections: 'Serious Games I, Watson is Down'; 'Serious Games II, Three Dead'; 'Serious Games III, Immersion'; and 'Serious Games IV, A Sun without Shadow'. All are split-screen, bar 'Serious Games II' which is a single-screen projection, and all are approximately eight minutes long, bar *Immersion*, which is approximately twenty minutes' duration

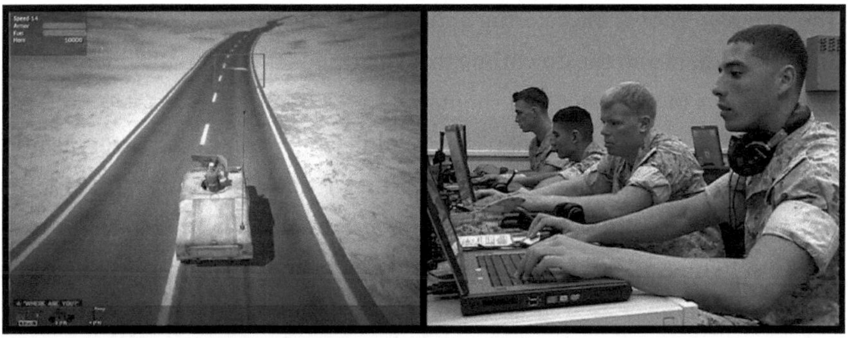

Figure 3.1 Harun Farocki, *Serious Games (I–IV)*, 2010. Serious Games I: Watson is Down, Video (colour, sound) 8 min. Courtesy HARUN FAROCKI FILMPRODUKTION and Greene Naftali, New York.

and is the film I shall mostly focus on due to its overtly pharmacological ethos. Filmed at the Marine Corps Base 29 Palms in California, 'Serious Games I, Watson is Down' shows four marines in a classroom being trained to shoot targets using a virtual imaging programme called 'Immersive Infantry Trainer'.[10] The four marines, representing the crew of a tank, sit in front of the laptop screens, using a mouse to steer their vehicle through a simulated landscape based on geographical data of Afghanistan. The programme involves the placement by the class instructor of explosive devices and insurgents in the area, which the soldiers learn to recognize and detonate in virtual game time. The viewer witnesses the virtual 'attacks' on the left-hand side of the screen, while the classroom is mainly shown on the right-hand side. The frontal format of the technology based on computer games gives the viewer the same view that the marines have on their screens. The effect is chilling. Is this really how young men learn how to navigate deadly weapons and make decisions to kill or not? 'Serious Games II, Three Dead' is also set on the 29 Palms base and documents a military manoeuvre in the fabricated Afghan city in the desert that is used for simulated military exercises in real time. The city buildings were made from containers whose flatness makes them look as if Farocki's team modelled them on a computer animation, a further slippage between realms of digital and real in the installation as a whole. The filmed 'event' shows around 300 extras, representing both the Afghan and Iraqi population, involved in an emergency manoeuvre in which a few dozen Marines go out on patrol to control a bomb threat and sniper fire.

The film also shows the catering and other facilities provided for the extras and the soldiers and the downtime that surrounds the 'dramatic' manoeuvre, as if it were a blockbuster film shoot.

'Serious Games III, Immersion' is filmed at Fort Louis, near Seattle, during a demonstration of VRET (Virtual Reality Exposure Therapy), a technology currently being patented for use by military therapists to treat PTSD sufferers.[11] VRET, which has had some minor success in alleviating a range of phobias as well as anorexia nervosa, consists of subjecting the patient to a virtual simulation that replicates the environment of their 'trauma'. The premise underlying this technological technique could be said to echo late nineteenth- and early twentieth-century discourses of hypnosis in psychology and psychoanalysis, e.g. Pierre Janet's notion that the imaginary re-enactment of traumatic events under hypnosis would liberate patients from their symptoms. However, in VRET, rather than the internal mental image generated under hypnosis, the image is an external projection that can be seen and manipulated by the therapist. This raises some concern. As Ruth Leys remarks in her masterful *Trauma: A Genealogy* (2000), Janet's emphasis on the productive nature of dissociation in hypnosis links to the emphasis in

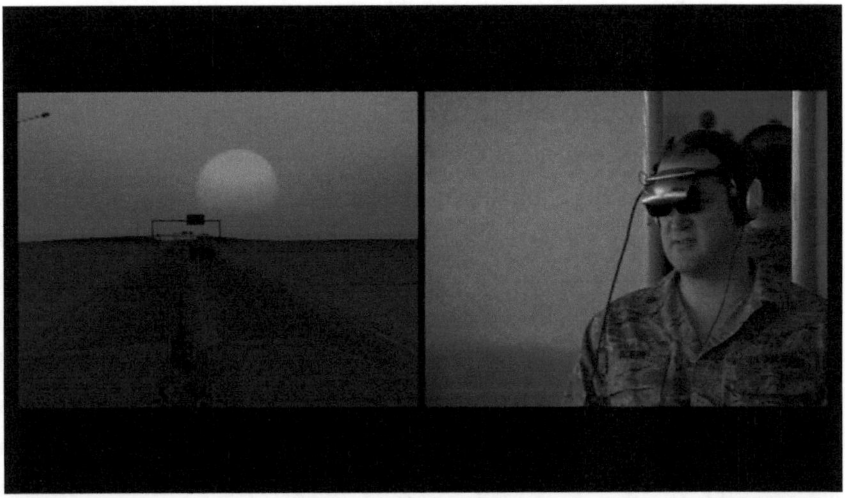

Figure 3.2 Harun Farocki, *Serious Games (I–IV)*, 2010. Serious Games III: Immersion (2009), Video (colour, sound) 20 min. Courtesy HARUN FAROCKI FILMPRODUKTION and Greene Naftali, New York.

contemporary neuropsychology on the embodied and adaptable brain whose negative thoughts and feelings can be modified by direct neuro-psychological intervention.[12]

In his discussion of *Serious Games*, cultural critic Pasi Väliaho makes a critical comparison between VRET and the hypno-cathartic therapies of sociologist George Simmel and Janet (2014: 74).[13] For Väliaho, unlike the latter's imaginary simulations of traumatic past events by patients drawn back to 'their unconscious memories and images [...] as well as the subjectively lived affective charges related to them' (74), in VRET, the PTSD sufferer's memories are not unconscious in this topological mental sense. In coupling users directly to their own physiological states, VR 'almost completely abolishes distinctions between internal and external worlds, between perception and image' (74) that Väliaho sees as necessary to integrating traumatic experience. For him, Virtual Iraq 'implements the suicidal logic of biopolitics, repeatedly reproducing the trauma of PTSD patients and accelerating the fears that it animates' (87). He sees this as capitalizing on neuroscientific knowledge about the reptilian part of the brain that involves the primitive drives of hunger, thirst, sexuality and territoriality and is dominated by fear and aggression. Replicating the logic of neoliberal subjectivity, which is to be in a 'self-perpetuating state of crisis', Väliaho claims that programmes such as Virtual Iraq inflict a fight or flight response that targets and attempts to rewire the 'reptilian parts of the brain' (80), training the amygdala to deal with aggressivity by harnessing it to technological instruments that ready for more violence. The impetus of this argument is that interventions such as VRET may 'cure' only by rechannelling the anger one might feel towards the toxic cause of the trauma, in this case, war, in the direction of a readiness to reengage. The lineage of the VRET technology we see being demonstrated in *Immersion* lends credence to Väliaho's critique, yet, in my encounter with Farocki's film, I want to persist with a more affirmative mode of therapeutic exorcism that does not deny the toxicity of the technology. Even Farocki states that in *Serious Games* he wanted to show how the artificial imagery of computer games technology is 'used *constructively* in ways that go beyond self-contained fictional universes' (Farocki in Ten Brink and Oppenheimer, 2012: 63, my emphasis).

Performative toxicity as cure

Virtual Iraq is based on a VR technology that, initially developed by the military, was subsequently taken over by game designers and marketed as Full Spectrum Warrior, a video game from 2004. Graphic elements from Full Spectrum Warrior have been recycled and redeveloped into the software program Virtual Iraq by clinical psychologist Skip Rizzo. This complete immersion in the military-industrial complex makes the programme's aims open to question. Adding to this suspicion, *Immersion* opens with Rizzo demonstrating the software programme, showing how its colour and density can be modulated in accordance with a patient's needs. As he adjusts the image gradation, Rizzo explains that dull grey is the best light to replicate 'the light of the traumatic experience', as if this is all it takes. The film continues by juxtaposing shots of therapists operating the programme on one side of the screen, while the second screen shows a number of 'soldiers' volunteering to wear the headset and act out traumatic war incidents which are simulated by the programme. Close-ups of the simulations they view through the headset often supplant the shots of the therapists operating the technology. The participants – three male and one female – change over quite rapidly until the final session lasting a good five minutes in which the 'soldier' wearing the headset becomes increasingly upset during the virtual re-enactment. The viewer interfaces intimately with his enactment as the jerky movements of the simulation shown on the left-hand side of the screen echo the soldier's head movements as he describes what happened on the day of the attack. As the soldier describes closing in on the kill, he feels increasingly sick. His verbal responses become increasingly dramatic. He sweats and appears about to vomit, reaching for a nearby bucket. The therapist tells him to keep going. 'You're doing a great job', she says. It is upsetting to watch, but also there is an air of expectancy. Are we going to witness a miracle cure in which the 'soldier' masters his traumatic experience and is relieved of his symptoms?

Suddenly, and almost imperceptibly, the image shifts from being a document of a 'therapy' session to being one of a performance. As the 'soldier' reaches the climactic threat of vomiting, he puts down the bucket saying, 'Some of that was real'. This is followed by the sound of clapping and the therapist standing up to explain the product's development. Gallery viewers begin to realize that what they have witnessed is a demonstration to market the value of VRET to the military. There is nothing to indicate this until the final unexpected moment when what one initially thinks is a bird's-eye view of reality reveals its performativity. As it turns out, the 'soldiers' are all military personnel, some of whom are therapists who work with soldiers suffering from PTSD. The therapist in the film was actually a former patient, the distressed soldier, a therapist.

On the one hand, Farocki's exposure of the commerce involved in this performance directs the viewer to mistrust the therapeutic scenario they have just witnessed and to perhaps formulate a critical attitude towards the technology in this context. This is underscored by Farocki in 'Serious Games IV, A Sun without Shadow', in which he makes a comparison between two sets of images,[14] juxtaposing them on the split screen. Moving away from the purely observational, the left-hand side of the screen presents the sardonic intertitle that the therapy programme is cheaper than the training programme as it does not render shadows, while, on the right-hand side, the desert townscape is rendered without shadow textures. In this part of *Serious Games*, Farocki takes up a critical position which feeds into Väliaho's reading that the 'soft montage' of the intertitles 'reflects back on its observer', asking us to question and evaluate the images we see (88). However, Farocki also professes to be interested by the 'symbolical generosity' of the virtual imaging technology which potentially enables war veterans to be rehabilitated in a social programme that shows that society has not forgotten what they have

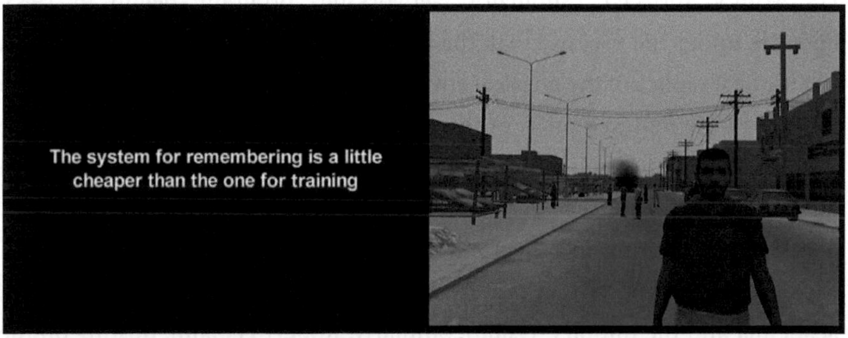

Figure 3.3 Harun Farocki, *Serious Games (I–IV)*, 2010. Serious Games IV: A Sun With No Shadow, Video (colour, sound). Courtesy HARUN FAROCKI FILMPRODUKTION and Greene Naftali, New York.

done (Farocki in Eshun, 2012: 76). I would say that this ambivalence is also embedded within the film. The performative re-enactment of traumatic war experience in *Immersion* inadvertently introduces the idea that a curative dimension might operate through what Stiegler calls a tertiary industrial projection, i.e. the technological exteriority of a medium that grounds the formation of primary and secondary memory. Rather than the reintegration of traumatic experience (Väliaho) or the exorcism of traumatic memory (Janet), a tertiary industrial projection, in this case, the virtual simulation, transmutes trauma beyond the individual's memory.

Unlike more phenomenologically oriented philosophy in which perception is originary, for Stiegler, primary perception and the secondary mnemonic retentions that are constructed from the former are both already propped on the tertiary modes of recording devices or transgenerational modes of transmission that are external to the subject. Applying Stiegler's argument, I propose that VRET, as shown in Farocki's film, acts as such a tertiary projection that enables traumatic experience to be environmentally narrated. Given its relation to the industrial-military-image complex, the resingularization or reindividuation of technical images that Stiegler calls for would seem to be impossible in *Serious Games*. However, for me, the film goes beyond the purely critical vein that Väliaho situates it within. Rather than presuming that immersive exposure to the site of traumatic memory accelerates symptoms as Väliaho suggests, might not this redoubling of life-at-a-distance create instead a kind of protective immunity necessary to the survivance of trauma?[15]

In her discussion of *Serious Games*, Sara Brady points out that the US Army's SIMNET (Simulator Networking) program, begun in 1983, operates under the premise that 'the best simulation training would provide, not the best replica of the physical environment of military operations, but the most accurate representation of the circumstances necessary to train for the *mental* capacity to function in the war theatre' (2016: 195). Further articles on VRET and its use to treat war trauma also point to its manipulative aspects. Sue Halpern, writing in *New Yorker*, refers to the partnerships involved in the development of Virtual Iraq as 'an unholy alliance between Hollywood, academia and the military' (2008). Similarly, Robert Hanafin, posting on the website Veterans Today, while not dismissing the technology out of hand, raises questions about the financial beneficiaries of 'imaginal therapy' (VRET) and the contracts between research and government, especially given that similar video games are readily available at Walmart (Hanafin, 2010). However, the various research papers that I accessed online, admittedly without being able to verify who funded them, tend to concur that: 'Preliminary data suggest that VRET is as efficacious as traditional exposure treatment and can be especially useful in the treatment of patients who are resistant to traditional exposure' (Gonçalves et al., 2012). The predominant view is that immersion in VR allows such patients to tolerate anxiety more easily, thereby overcoming their avoidance of (verbal) triggers in traditional exposure therapy such as CBT (Nijdam and Vermetten, 2018).[16] Underscoring the psychical economy of this technology, Brady cites Rizzo:

> VRET offers a way to circumvent the natural avoidance tendency by directly delivering multi-sensory and context-relevant cues that evoke the trauma without demanding that the patient actively try to access his/her experience through effortful memory retrieval. (Rizzo in Brady, 2012: 98)

Evaluating the efficacy of this therapeutic technology is beyond my expertise, but what I'm interested in here is its imaginary potential, as presented in *Serious Games*, to work by exacerbating anxiety, on the one hand, and projecting 'memory' beyond the individual, on the other. As an aesthetic modality, the former counters the benign nature of therapeutic mindfulness cultures in cognitive capitalism that advocate making a friend of anxiety, i.e. suppressing it. And the performative projection of memory-at-a-distance is suggestive of a process in which the virtual image might potentially enable a sufferer to bear anxiety without having to assume the position of moral strength in which cure is equivalent to self-will. The image-apparatus bears the burden, exteriorizing it so that a sufferer can find some relief from feeling that they are to blame for their symptoms. In this transitional environment, Stiegler's tertiary projection, rather than rewiring the reptilian brain, might enable a recasting of the boundary between inner and outer reality. In offering patients a simulated control over experiences that haunt them, VRET, as a transitional space of projection, could be said to enable these experiences to be cathected at-a-distance, thereby relieving the sufferer from the supposed responsibility of failing to integrate them into their psyche. If PTSD is characterized by the dissociation between experience and memory, the interest of VRET for my developing argument is that, as an aesthetic treatment in Farocki's film, the simulation, the image-at-a-distance, comes to stand in for the event of memory and so enable a perspective on it. Admittedly, I am conflicted about speculating from my encounter with *Immersion* (and various theoretical texts) about the therapeutic aesthetics of a technology that issues from the military-industrial complex. But, in order to survive well without denying the toxicity of life-limiting and harmful situations, I would maintain with Brady, in her discussion of *Serious Games*, that 'play is perhaps the only way out of an experience that is similarly *not* play' (Brady, 2016: 200).

Farocki has also intimated the importance of role-play in relation to the 'symbolical generosity' of the programme. In a discussion between Farocki and Kodwo Eshun, Eshun explicitly articulates the pharmacological nature of the work:

> [I]t's clear that the project as such is to study a way in which the image comes with the claim to both inflict harm and then to repair that harm. The dialectic of the contemporary image, and the way in which the image holds out a promise of curing the havoc that it creates. [. . .] the military can't possibly think that the image that creates harm is also the image that will cure that harm. (Eshun, 2012: 72)

Farocki responds by talking about the imaginative, rather than manipulative, power of role-play documented in the work. The fact that a manipulated computerized image stands-in for and perhaps replaces a 'real' experience and that a manufactured performance stands-in for a moment of cathartic discharge does not overrule the 'symbolical generosity' that might operate in the transitional environment of the film. Such a pharmacological aesthetic seems more applicable to a digital age in which the Freudian characterization of the unconscious as the repressed has less currency than the idea of the unconscious as performative; it acts rather than represents (Leys, 2000: 267).[17]

Something of this performativity can also be seen in a work by artists Larry Achiampong and David Blandy *FF Gaiden: Control* (2016). This is one of the series of works under the FF Gaiden title, which use the video game *Grand Theft Auto V* to engage different communities to narrate traumatic or difficult personal experiences. For *FF Gaiden: Control*, the artists worked with veterans in Her Majesty's Prison in Althouse and Liverpool, the project being commissioned by FACT Liverpool as part of the Veterans in Practice programme to include a part of the ex-Forces community that it had previously neglected, i.e. those who are in prison due to difficulties adjusting to civilian life often as a result of PTSD.[18] Obtaining permission to bring PlayStation 4s into the category B prisons, the games (with violent content removed) formed a virtual world in which a group of prisoners and some family members could explore their own traumatic experiences through an avatar of their choosing. This was not therapy in the strict sense, the voice-over narrations in the resulting gallery film ranging from poems to reflections on childhood and adolescence, social control, violence and abuse, as well as hope for the future. As Blandy puts it:

> Exploration of the seemingly limitless virtual space of GTA5 from inside the prison seemed to open up ideas and possibilities for the participants, as did the possibility of self-transformation through their choice of avatar. The Avatar also acted as a mask, enabling an openness of expression. So it both enabled and deepened our conversations, the process engendering a trust that resulted in the work.[19]

Watching *FF Gaiden: Control* relieves the viewer from judging or identifying with the participants, as one hypnotically follows the various avatars who, beginning underwater, move through cityscapes and over vast mountainous terrain, the repetitious continuity of their journeys removing the heroism associated with reaching sublime peaks and overcoming obstacles. The altered video game serves as a vehicle not to return prisoners to the site of trauma or to give viewers a bird's-eye view of another's traumatic experience, but to allow memory to move in ways that are both uninhibited and constrained in conjunction with the virtual landscape. Although at a ground level, the narrated experiences are very much owned by the participants, as they are enfolded into the virtual image operating as a mode of tertiary projection, they become loosened from particular bodies so that gallery viewers too can enfold themselves into these traumatic experiences without ascribing pity or denial. The avatar as mask facilitates this, the altered game-scape becoming a tool that enables memories to be both disassociated from the traumatic event per se and processed at-a-distance without interpretation. It supplies the illusion necessary to this process, the transitional space of illusion being what is killed off by the extremely powerful hormones and stress reactors of PTSD that render individuals powerless. The videogame space, devoid of its usual goal-oriented drivers, provides the imaginative space of tertiary projection that, in facilitating role-play, enables a potential resingularization of traumatic memory that is shared socially.

It might at this point sound far-fetched to propose that performative, rather than interactive, demonstrations of such virtual environments in the gallery might also be a useful treatment for viewers whose feelings of powerlessness in relation to global phenomena such as war and systemic violence make them feel hopeless and depressed. But this notion is what I shall develop differently in future chapters. For now I will conclude that rather than offering a model of how things should be or what we can do about things, the pharmacological aesthetics of works such as *Serious Games* and *FF Gaiden: Control* involves the creation of transitional spaces in which the irresolvable dichotomy of poison and cure can be imagined and engaged with without denying either side of the divide. And this affordance of ambivalence is liberating in a socio-economic order that, in its quantification of both psychic and social life, only encourages and rewards the performance of positivity.

4

Homeopathic mimicry in Omer Fast's war trilogy

In this chapter, I shall explore Omer Fast's war-themed gallery film installations in relation to Steven Shaviro's notion of 'homeopathic magic' (2010: 23). Shaviro's concept relates to the pharmacological aesthetics of how poison and cure are imbricated in one and the same substance and how this can be applied in aesthetic productions in a neoliberal cognitive capitalist context. While Shaviro prefers to use the terms 'global' or 'late capitalism', his idea is that its sicknesses (poisons) can only be treated in art and filmworks by a homeopathic mimicry of the same kinds of sickness. This filmic doubling has curative potential in providing the viewer with a sense of survival that can be linked to the inoculation effects of Benjamin's anaesthetics that I referred to in Chapter 2. While the media works that Shaviro addresses in *Post Cinematic Affect*, i.e. from a digital music video to mainstream films that emulate gamespace, are different from my artists' moving image case studies, contemporary media ecology can be said to be characterized by an aesthetics in which hybrid spaces derived from television, video and digital media clash. Hence Shaviro's use of the term 'post-cinematic media regime' (87). However rather than simply applying Shaviro's notion of homeopathic magic or mimicry, my aim is to explore how technical images can be used by a range of actors, i.e. pro- and post-filmic participants including audiences, as a life-enhancing mechanism of inoculation. To make my case, I will contrast Fast's work on war trauma with Krzysztof Wodiczko's *Abraham Lincoln: War Veteran Projection, Union Square* (2012), a public art image-sound piece in which the upper torsos of a number of veterans suffering from PTSD were projected onto Lincoln's statue from where they are heard speaking their trauma. As opposed to the overtly therapeutic impetus of Wodiczko's work that uses art as a means of consciousness-raising, Fast's war-themed narratives immerse their viewers in traumatic symptomatology through imaginative role-play. Rather than the coolness of Farocki's immanent critique that looks dispassionately at the documented environment, in Fast's mode of 'homeopathic magic', critique becomes as exploitative and sick as that which it documents or mirrors. But, paradoxically, in this sickness, there is hope of transformation.

I had long admired Fast's use of film in the gallery to create spatialized fictions that fluently mash and borrow from various cinematic genres to speak to contemporary issues of psychological trauma, migration and war, but, in terms of researching for this book, I was particularly struck by audience responses to an artists' talk he gave at the Imperial War Museum in 2013 on the occasion of the museum's exhibition of *5000 Feet is the Best*.[1] At the talk, Fast showed extracts from *The Casting* (2007) and *Continuity* (2012), which, along with *5000 Feet is the Best* (2011), can loosely be referred to as a war trilogy. Although I shall not discuss it at great length here, *Continuity* was particularly compelling in its mirroring of the sickness of war by an analogously perverse domestic narrative. The looped film comprises sequences in which a bourgeois middle-aged couple repeatedly drive to a bus stop to pick up a different young man in combat uniform. The first time one witnesses the scene, whether this be the first sequence or a later sequence depending on one's entry to the installation, one might surmise that this is a soldier returning from duty to visit his parents. But once the 'family' arrive home, the sexual inferences between them troubles this idea, suggesting either that the couple's compulsive routine is a dissociative way of dealing with the traumatic loss of a son killed in the Iraq War or that they are simply perverse and have a penchant for hiring male prostitutes to engage in role-play. Either way, the film turns the tables on the familiar scenario of returning home from war which is usually represented as heroism or victimhood. Seeing the father character, played by André Hennicke, sticking his tongue inside the mouth of the returning soldier 'son' in his bedroom jolts the viewer out of such identificatory tropes.

For me the work operated as an analogous mirroring of the perversity of war, driving home the point that war is itself a perverse form of statecraft. Fast seemed to have found a novel strategy for representing this theatre, not by documenting it or making a docu-fiction, but by creating a fictional narrative that brought its criminal underbelly home, so to speak. One might ask, how is this effective, it doesn't change anything? But this would be to miss the function of art which is not necessarily to raise consciousness or offer solutions but to enable us to engage, in this case, with the horror and trauma of war, without being overwhelmed by empathy or dismissive through compassion fatigue. Fast's therapeutic aesthetics counters the propagandistic tenor of mainstream cinematic representations of war that advocate heroism or victimhood by inventing a 'sick', yet equally seductive, story.

The audience response to Fast's talk and presentation of his films was telling. No one questioned the artist. Everyone was polite, but in the exit queues, I was surrounded by people from different age groups and walks of life complaining how disgusting the work was and how sick the artist must be. While the Imperial War Museum has an educational remit, it is nonetheless a memorial to the war effort and its artefacts. Its displays honour war and its technologies, making them available for family viewing and remembrance. Fast's work seemed to be undermining the sacrificial heroism and the symbolism of war paraphernalia which maintain war as a form of patriotism rather than a criminal act. Added to this, his fictional manipulation of his interviews with real soldiers and, in *5000 Feet is the Best*, an ex-drone operator suffering from post-traumatic symptoms, can be considered exploitative. However, my point is that his use of fiction not only admits to the manipulative elements of moving image per se, but also mirrors how exploitation operates in neoliberal cognitive capitalism more generally. In this his work acts as a poisonous remedy, a pharmakon.

Fast's trilogy of war films are not *about* soldiers or drone operators but *about* how audiences of mediated representations of war might engage with trauma in a mode of fabulation that counters the compassion fatigue that often arises in relation to TV news and related documentary reportage. T.J. Demos suggests that Fast's work performs a retooling of 'media and the technological conventions of storytelling in order to invent new possibilities for meaningful aesthetic forms […] and interpretive agency appropriate to our own age' (Demos, 2012: 84). Citing Virilio, Demos characterizes this as one in which we have moved beyond the deferred time 'of historical thought, literary expression, and reflective analysis– into the "real time" of the electronic screen, satellite electronics and the total flow of video imagery' (Demos, 2012: 83).

Demos is here obliquely referencing Cathy Caruth's notion of history as a form of traumatic deferral.[2] Whereas, as I discussed in the previous chapter, and more in line with 'the total flow of video imagery', trauma is currently used to describe the general logic of neoliberal subjectivity as a condition of being in a 'self-perpetuating state of crisis' (Väliaho, 2014: 85). This state is characterized by an all-pervasive and immediate sense of anxiety that stems from living in an era of constant catastrophes, or threat of catastrophe, whether large or small. The challenge for artists, especially those working with moving image which is intimately connected to the entertainment-industrial complex, is to find ways of expressing this crisis without being subsumed by it.

Fast's faux-analytic settings in *5000 Feet is the Best* and *The Casting* involve a fictional exacerbation of traumatic symptomatology which I align with Shaviro's notion that it is only artworks that are fully ensconced in the flows of capital and its violence that are up to the task of telling us something about it, of making its abstractions real. Shaviro's view is that films and artworks that narrate the catastrophic subjectivities that result from global capitalism might, by showing us subjects who are both traumatized by and able to manipulate conditions of extreme precarity, act as allegories of survivance. I shall argue that such a therapeutic aesthetic does not 'cure' but provides the inoculating effect necessary to what Judith Butler calls a mode of productive 'living on' that does not yield fully repaired humans.[3]

The Casting

Fast's initial idea for *The Casting* was to film the Fort Irwin military base in the Mohave desert, a training centre which, akin to the one used in Farocki's 'Serious Games II: Three Dead', uses 3-D simulations of Iraqi villages inhabited by extras from the local community to prepare soldiers for war. While waiting to get a permit to film, which was eventually refused, he went to Fort Hood in Texas and interviewed soldiers who had undergone the training and then experienced their first tour in Iraq. Rather than using the soldier's stories first hand, Fast wanted 'to include a measure of the mediation that happens to their stories and the kind of forces, interests and desires that act upon them as they become a public narrative art piece' (Fast in Simblist, 2012).

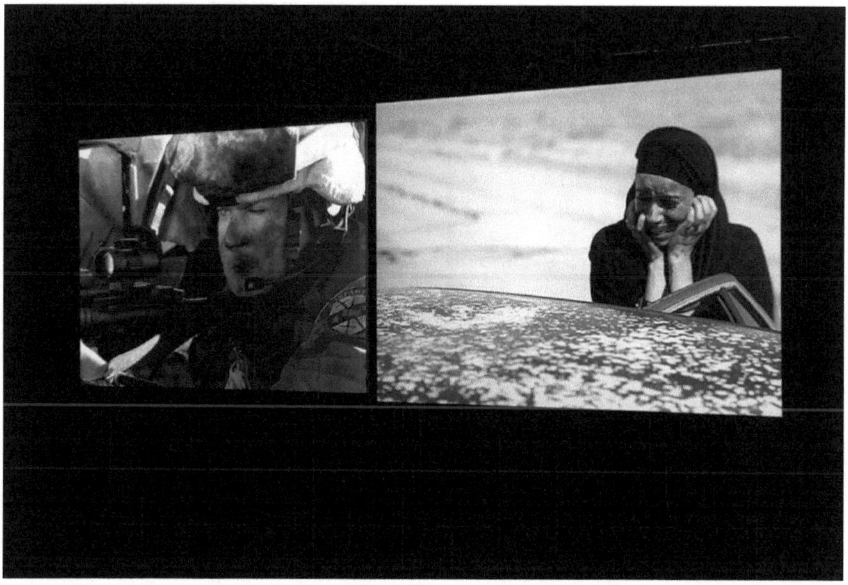

Figure 4.1 Omer Fast, *The Casting*, 2007. Four-channel video installation, colour, sound, duration: 14 minutes, Credit: Nick Trikonis, Courtesy of the artist and James Cohan, New York.

The installation consists of a double-sided projection, each side featuring a split screen.[4] The dual screen facing the viewer as they enter the gallery presents a series of shots depicting three different but interrelated locations: a casting studio where a director, a stand-in perhaps for Fast, auditions an actor to play a soldier in a film; and a soldier's tour of duty in Iraq which in turn is intercut with a story about his time being stationed at a military base in Germany. All the shots in the film are static, the actors' gestures being held still in a manner reminiscent of the tableaux vivantes in primitive cinema. The film begins with a fast-paced montage of the audition, Fast's voice-over posing the question: 'How do you feel about improvising? So, let's improvise'. Initially, the viewer is perhaps unaware that the voice-over narration, which seems like a continuous monologue, relates to the back projection, whose split screen shows two talking heads: Fast himself on one side and, on the adjacent side, an actor standing in for a soldier suffering from PTSD. The actor's answer to Fast's questions provides the voice-over narration to the front projections. Unlike the close synchronization between the images on the front screens and the apparent continuity of this narration, the back side 'documentary'

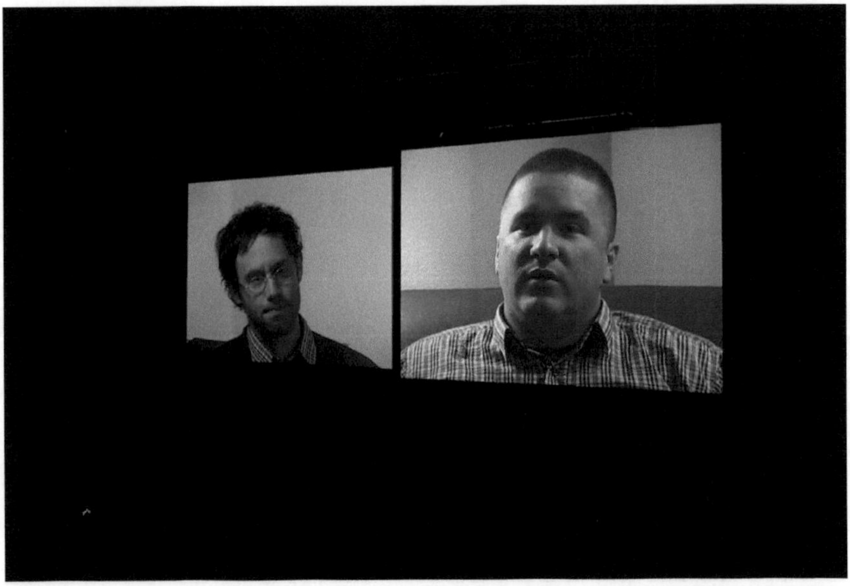

Figure 4.2 Omer Fast, *The Casting* 2007. Four-channel video installation, colour, sound. Duration: 14 minutes, Credit: Nick Trikonis, Courtesy of the artist and James Cohan, New York.

images of Fast and the actor soldier are sharply cut. Their clothes change in the middle of sentences at unpredictable intervals, underscoring the fabrication of the narrative script's seamlessness and undermining the documentary truth effects of the simulated interview.

The auditioning actor's monologue recounts a story about being stationed in Germany and meeting a neurotic self-harming German girl who invites him to spend Christmas with her and her family. Shots showing the characters of this story are rapidly intercut with shots showing the soldier with his team beside a military airplane in 'Iraq', with shots of the studio being intermittently inserted. Sometimes both screens show the same locations, sometimes the locations are juxtaposed, the changeover from one scene to the next often occurring after the use of trigger words in the voice-over narration. For example, the word 'driving' appears to trigger a shift from shots of being in his girlfriend's car in Germany to riding in a Humvee in Iraq; the word 'there' seems to prompt a shift from Germany to the military base in Iraq; 'burn' segues from close-ups of the girlfriend's scars due to self-harm to scenes of a hot desert and the 'fireball' that woke the soldier out of his stupor while on patrol in the Humvee. Believing that his team are under threat, the soldier accidentally shoots an unarmed Iraqi male civilian who was in the back seat of a car that refused to stop. A sequence of static shots show the man's family pulling his bloody body from the vehicle, followed by a close-up of his wife's face, framed by her blood-covered hands, her scream silently posed, creating the kind of suspension effect reminiscent of what Gilles Deleuze calls an 'affection-image', i.e. an image suspended between perception and action. (It also reminds me of the infamous still of the screaming nurse from Sergei Eisenstein's *Battleship Potemkin* (1925).) For Patricia Pisters, the affection-image has the ability to 'touch us in a direct and embodied way [and] speak directly to the spectators feeling of empathy' (Pisters in Martin, 2017: 79). However, in Fast's mode of what he calls 'trauma-turned-drama' (Fast in Fiduccia, 2008: 158), the awkwardness of these suspended actions unsettles the empathetic identification between spectators and characters and formally mimics the dissociative representation of traumatic experience. How so?

One of Fast's sources of reference in making this work was Susan Sontag's *Regarding the Pain of Others*. Acknowledging that it is not possible, or perhaps ethical, to represent the horror of what the soldiers had experienced, he proposes instead what he calls

> a game of substitution. [. . .] instead of substituting the pathos of the soldier's story with the pathos of actors acting, I'm going to give you to the pathos of the body under duress. The director commands the body to freeze but the body is breathing and twitching at the moment you want it to be still. (Fast in Verhagen, 2009: 4)

While the technique of instructing his actors to freeze derived in part from Fast's anxiety about directing actors,[5] the result disallows the viewer's assimilation of the other, either the soldier or those he harms, thereby making it difficult to identify a victim or a perpetrator to pity or revile. Teasing the viewer with the tropes of narrative identification – characters, family romance, a crime – Fast makes them hard to fully invest in.

In her appraisal of this film, Erika Balsom is critical of Fast's use of continuity editing, seeing it as unquestioning of the conventional codes of mainstream cinema. As she describes it: 'When a character speaks via voice-over, the image track cuts in for a medium close-up and shot/reverse-shot depicting the conversational exchange' (2013: 149) which is emitting from the back side of the projection.[6] For Balsom, Fast empties the soldiers' words 'of any attestation to the real [...] negating the referential power of the documentary image and placing it on the same plane as fiction' (Balsom, 2013: 153). However, not only is this the point, but also, truth-telling in documentary, especially in relation to the recounting of traumatic memory, is itself subject to falsification or confabulation.[7] To remember is a process of bringing memory into being, of constructing it. It is, as I referred to it in the introduction, a pharmakon in which the fictional and the real cannot be divorced as experience is always reliant on and constituted in relation to mediation. Fast's multivalent narrative performs the construction of memory. Highlighting its own staginess, the film asks the question of what it is we are doing when we identify with another's trauma. Rather than assimilating 'the other's experience to the self' which Jill Bennett, following Brecht, refers to as 'crude empathy' (Bennett 2005: 10), Fast's awkward freezing of his actors' poses creates a space in which we might test out the positionalities of self and other: who is the perpetrator, who is the victim; why do some have the right to speak, while others are silenced? However, this is not simply critique. While Fast identifies his interest in 'processes of defamiliarization, from the uncanny to the Brechtian' (in Vinyes Albes 2015: 107),[8] he is not interested in either manipulation or in supposedly critiquing the media, but in pleasure as a means to master trauma. Referring to Brechtian analyses, he says:

> Of course these critical analyses have been important in fashioning our understanding of the media but I think all that talk tends to obscure something which is extremely important in the media and that is pleasure. [...] I want to make things that are pleasurable, regardless of their relationship to social dynamics and to current events, to history and the media. (in Verhagen: 2009: 2)

This might sound flippant, but it can also be considered as a pharmacological approach to the representation of trauma, one that denies neither the inherent toxicity of mediation nor its remedial capacity to transmit experience. Fast's transmission of traumatic experience across the time and space of the interlinked stories shifts 'the burden of sorting through the traumatic event [...] along to the viewer as the event is visibly transformed into a public performance' (Fast in Fiduccia, 2008: 158). In such a filmic transitional space, traumatic symptomatology shifts from being a personal attachment to an originary event and becomes a performative arena in which characters, actors and viewers become co-conspirators in stories that uncoil repetition from being a repetition of the same, i.e. an inhibitory repetition. This is not a total healing but, as Susan Buck-Morss says: 'repetition is never merely repetition. There is always something new in the experience as well – which is why it is possible to be healed of a trauma' (in Kester, 1997: 45).

While I am not interested in psychoanalyzing artists or tracing the 'truth' of their work in their autobiographies, Fast's interest in traumatic memory and his irreverent play with it are surely not unrelated to his Israeli ethnicity and generational distance to the Holocaust – he was born in 1972. He grew up in Israel and New York and for him '[t]his idea of trauma, its presence and absence, the way it reverberates in time and in a community is something that I grew up with on both sides of that ocean' (Fast in Simblist, 2012). It is also noteworthy that his earlier two-channel video *Spielberg's List* (2003) exemplifies this trauma-at-a-distance, in relation to not only geographical and temporal locations but also the use of media images in the construction of memory.[9] *Spielberg's List* consists of footage of documentary-style talking heads interviews of the extras from Spielberg's *Schindler's List* (1993), which was filmed on location in Krakow using extras from the local population. This material is mixed with footage showing remnants of the real camps as well as Spielberg's sets, which, now falling to ruin, have become a tourist attraction in the area. As the interviews progress, the extras clearly begin to confuse their memories of the Holocaust with their re-enactment of it in Spielberg's film. The construction of memory does not easily distinguish between classes of images, the real and its media representation becoming equally virtual, the boundary between them unstable. While this lack of definitive distinction may seem somewhat alarming, it is important to note that history is not simply a recounting of facts but a method of ordering events that are deemed worthy of remembrance, such recording systems and their values changing over time. Rather than 'truth', Fast plays with forms and layers of mediation in imagining 'how a traumatic experience travels, the way that it ripples out from its ground zero and its point of origin and how it passes through different bodies and different layers of bodies in a particular community' (Fast in Simblist, 2012). For me, Fast's performative staging of traumatic memory and creative distortion can be aligned with psychoanalyst Jean Laplanche's notion that as children we pick up the traces of our parents' unconscious desires without understanding them and this motivates us to fill in the gaps of our understanding by means of representation. Laplanche calls this gap, which is generative of symbolic play, the enigmatic signifier (1999).[10]

At this juncture, I want to throw my argument into relief by contrasting Fast's performative play with trauma to a well-intentioned work by Krzysztof Wodiczko, *Abraham Lincoln: War Veteran Projection, Union Square* (2012). This contrast underscores the difference between the pharmacological aesthetics I am pursuing and aesthetics as a branch of art therapy. *Abraham Lincoln: War Veteran Projection, Union Square* (2012) is a twenty-three-minute loop of talking head footage of fourteen war veterans, including some family members, projected onto Abraham Lincoln's memorial statue in Union Square Park. Superimposed over Lincoln's larger-than-life upper torso to uncanny effect, the veterans recount harrowing war experiences, speaking their trauma from a public site commemorating liberty. For this work, Wodiczko and his team worked for several months with New York City veterans' organizations and dozens of war veterans and their families, fourteen of whom stayed the course. It is hard not to be moved by the footage of Wodiczko's reanimation of the dead heroism of this public monument, making Lincoln's statue quite literally speak to commemorate the silenced narratives of recent war-at-a-distance and the psychological experience of damage that continues long after service is over. Projecting the testaments of war veterans, normally invisible to the general public, onto such a public monument is a very powerful restorative gesture which Wodiczko claims as overtly therapeutic. But is there a danger that in the process testimony is transformed into spectacle?

The work builds on Wodiczko's previous work using projections on public monuments. In *Krakow Town Hall* (1996), for example, he projected onto the building's main central tower larger-than-life footage of inhabitants of Krakow speaking of the problems and traumas they experience in the city, partly as a legacy of the Soviet regime. For him, the purpose of this work was to give voice to trauma in public space. He states that:

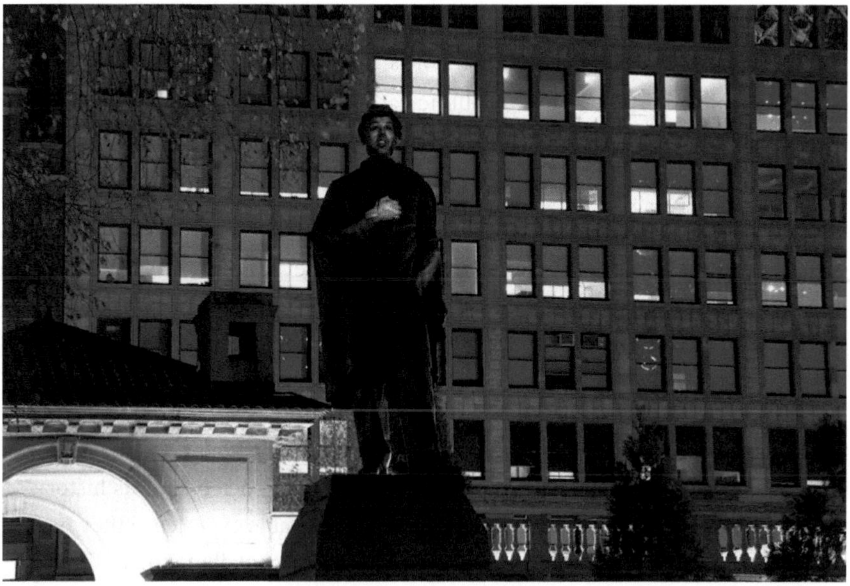

Figure 4.3 Krzysztof Wodiczko, *Abraham Lincoln: War Veteran Projection, Union Square, New York*, 2012. © Krzysztof Wodiczko. Courtesy Galerie Lelong & Co., New York.

> From silence to animation, the participant must become a speaking monument testifying in public and demanding larger change. This makes such a person psychologically healthier and socially useful for others while making the monument feel better and more useful as well. (Wodiczko in Beech, 2017: 4)

In the same interview, he also discusses earlier work from the 1970s made under Poland's oppressive conditions that were paradoxically supported by the regime, experimental media art, considered seemingly non-political, being used to enable its double-speak claim that it was not censorious. As Wodiczko says, 'the authorities needed high-quality media art knowledge and skills to secure the effectiveness of their media-run propaganda apparatus' (in Beech 2017: 1–2). Although the mode of governance and historical eras are different, nonetheless, a not dissimilar kind of double-speak could be said to be operative in relation to Wodiczko's *Abraham Lincoln*. For example, the licence given to Wodiczko for the use of the monument for his therapeutic intentions is disproportionate to the reduction in US government funding for rehabilitation programmes for war veterans. The lack of governmental aid for rehabilitation programmes is not my issue here, but whether, in projecting the veterans' faces and stories onto Lincoln's memorial statue, Wodiczko's work could be said to enact a kind of public catharsis that redeems the imperialist use of war as a means of global domination. As well as this, the media spectacle and its context of projection, a busy tourist site that encourages distracted viewing, could be said to allow audiences to recuperate these traumatic stories, situating the soldiers as 'not-me' others to be either ignored or shrouded with pity. But on the other hand, perhaps the work works differently for different recipients. As Wodiczko says in the Brooklyn Rail:

> Those veterans who saw themselves speaking this way in a public space and critically interpreting the world in which they live, may see themselves as being 'outside of themselves' and a part of larger society and its history. [...] By publicly telling the truth of their unacceptable experience they may inspire, develop, or reinforce their wish and will to contribute to new public consciousness toward the larger change—perhaps toward the future world free from wars and war veterans. Perhaps this is the aim of the kind of art I do? Not art therapy, but art that has a social, critical, and therapeutic effect and a psychoanalytic dimension. (in Ann McCoy, 2014)

Although I am swayed by Wodiczko's intentions to heal society, I also think that the work paradoxically runs the risk of engendering an overwhelming sense of grief and empathy that overrides the capacity for change. Sara Ahmed's reflections on how we consume the pain of others summarize my feeling of abject powerlessness in relation to the veterans' tragic stories. As Ahmed says:

> the pain of others becomes 'ours', an appropriation that transforms and neutralizes their pain into our sadness. It is not so much that we are 'with them' by feeling sad; the apparently shared negative feeling state does not position the reader and victim in a relation of equivalence. Rather, we feel sad *about* their suffering, an 'aboutness' that ensures that they remain the object of 'our feeling'. (Ahmed 2004: 35)

While it may have been therapeutic for the soldiers and their families who stayed the course to participate in the process,[11] the spectacle of the resulting projections in *Abraham Lincoln: War Veteran Projection, Union Square* runs the risk of engendering an empathetic sadness that may ultimately make the spectator feel good about themselves as worthy witnesses of another's testimony. On a panel, which included Wodiczko, called 'War, Trauma and Public Art' held in collaboration with New York University in 2012, Carl Cannon, a Vietnam veteran who participated in the project and works as Peer Counsellor for Services for the Underserved, stated that, while he was appreciative of Wodiczko's work, it is nonetheless a beautiful work of art whereas he is dealing with everyday suffering.[12] This statement unwittingly resonates with Leo Bersani's critique of the culture of redemption that salvages damaged experience by clothing it in a normative reparation that fails to acknowledge the destructive aspects involved in any reparative act (1990). Without this acknowledgement, cultural artefacts and works are at risk of becoming used for propagandistic purposes. While Wodiczko sees his work as part of an effort to end war – undoubtedly a social good but not one that art is going to bring about – Fast asserts that ethics are not particularly interesting criteria for judging or making a work of art (Fiduccia 2008: 173). His equally manipulative use of 'trauma-turned-drama' seems to me to acknowledge the entanglement of poison and cure in the representation of trauma whereas Wodiczko's well-intentioned work tries to separate them. Unlike the cool observational performativity of Farocki's *Serious Games*, yet paradoxically akin to its ethics, 'trauma-turned-drama' mimes the toxicity of fractured experience in global capitalism due to the traumatic effects of global warfare-at-a-distance.[13] In this mimicry, Fast puts the symptoms of post-traumatic experience to work in a way that does not seek to integrate it in a singular sufferer, an 'other', but to circulate it amongst a series of actors. He describes trauma-turned-drama as

> presenting the players that attend to it along the way as it transforms: from the individual at the outset – in this case the soldier turned interviewee – to the interviewer, the 'artist', and a larger public including the director, the crew and the actors. (in Fiduccia, 2008: 158)

Key to this circulation is the interweaving of the two stories in *The Casting* whereby 'the tragic inevitability of the one is intruded upon, perhaps sometimes stalled by the other' (in Fiduccia: 159). Montage here assembles, rather than cuts, a technique Janet Harbord calls 'editing as contagion' (2007: 80), a cinematic mode of linking different geo-spatial and temporal locations in which separate places and times coalesce. Such a mode of editing is an aesthetic response to the complexities of a globalized world.[14] Through the technique of montage as assemblage, traumatic or catastrophic experience becomes dispersed across a field of relations in a transitional space of confabulation.

5000 Feet is the Best

5000 Feet is the Best takes this to another level. The single-screen installation features an ex-drone operator suffering from PTSD who is being interviewed in a Las Vegas hotel. The actors, Gabriel Gutierrez, who plays the faux journalist/director, a stand-in for Fast, and Denis O'Hare, who plays the former drone operator now working as casino security, engage in a dialogue. The script is based on material gleaned from two actual interviews that Fast undertook with a real-life ex-drone operator suffering from PTSD, parts of which appear in a pixelated talking head sequence later in the film where the operator describes his 'work'. The staged interview is continually interrupted by bleeps, unheard by the interviewer, that trigger O'Hare's ex-drone operator character to go out into the corridor. On each of the three occasions he leaves the room, a different mini-narrative, voiced over by O'Hare, gets played out. The idea for this 'elusive and multivalent' structure (Fast in Simblist, 2012) came from the fact that the actual pilot was reluctant to discuss his experiences and became more open only on his frequent cigarette breaks, but in the film, the three mini-narratives function as confabulations that transform the dissociative symptomatology of PTSD into something potentially creative.

The first narrative sequence occurs after O'Hare goes out for a smoke and features a black-American man so obsessed by trains that he illegally drives one for a day. Strangely enough, O'Hare's character had bumped into this man in the hotel corridor at the very beginning of the film, each of the mini-narratives having an association with something that he perceives in the corridor as if the latter is a liminal dream space triggering fantasy. The train driver gets away with it, but, ironically, he is arrested by police for breaking into his own house after forgetting his keys. The interviewer asks why this man had to be black, to which O'Hare angrily responds: 'I didn't say anything about race', the final shots of this mini-narrative showing a younger white man being arrested, such substitutions and doubling being a feature of

Fast's work in general. The second mini-narrative features a male and female criminal team who scam male hotel guests; the woman seduces them in hotel bedrooms whose en-suite bathrooms are stocked with a range of men's trousers to replace the ones they lose when, caught in the act by her partner, they get thrown out of the room, the couple coveting the target's wallet. The third and longest sequence features a white bourgeois American family going for a trip in a homeland under occupation by an Asian military who check their papers on exiting the city. Unbeknownst to them, they enter a kill zone. A drone, its surveillance data in Asian characters, hovers over three white armed suspects, referred to as shepherds by the voice-over narration, suspiciously digging a hole at the side of a country road. The drone strikes, blowing up both vehicles and vaporizing the suspects, but the family emerge from their vehicle resurrected as zombies that walk off into the sunset in the manner of TV series such as *The Walking Dead*.

These three narrative sequences can be read as expressions of a psychic state of dissociation, the first two narratives coalescing around objects that are stolen and the idea of getting away with things before eventually being caught. In psychoanalytic theory, stealing is often a substitutive act to cover up or act out a traumatic experience, stealing being both a pointing to and a filling in

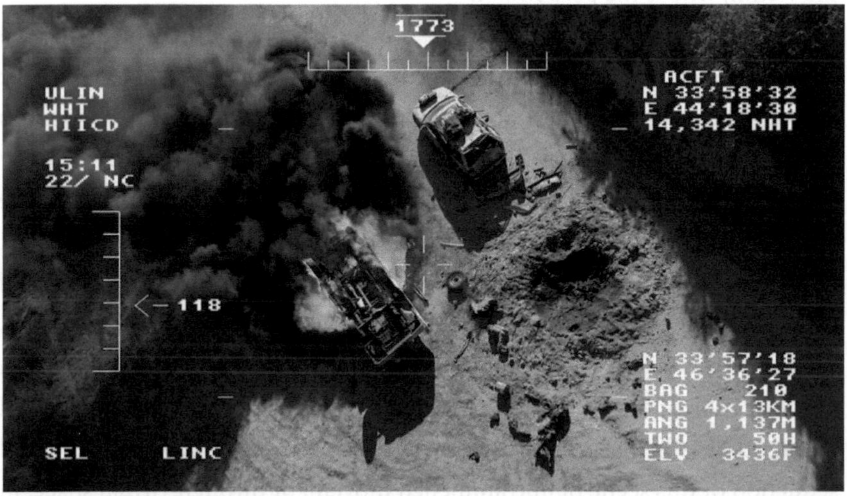

Figure 4.4 Omer Fast, *5000 Feet is the Best*, 2011. Single-channel HD video, colour, sound. Duration: 30 minutes looped, Credit: Nick Trikonis, Courtesy of the artist and James Cohan, New York.

of the absence of consciousness that is purported by Caruth and others to lie at the core of traumatic event(s).[15] However, unlike the psychoanalytic concept of trauma as repressed, in Fast's narrations, the traumatic event is performative. In being dispersed across spaces incorporating a multiplicity of protagonists, the irruptive time of trauma, a time characterized by aural and visual flashbacks and/or hallucinations, is transformed into a relay of scenes that restore the capacity of illusion that PTSD destroys. Fast's assembly of shots could be described as having three times: the time of an event in the past relayed by his interviewee; the time of the recording of the interview and filming of staged material; and the time of editing which assembles the first two times in such a way that they begin to break in on each other, passing information from one layer of time to the other. As well as this, Fast's substitutions blur the boundaries between categories of 'them' and 'us' that predominate in the imperialistic outsourcing of war to countries such as Iraq and Afghanistan on the justification that democracy is being secured for the victimized 'other'. The layering of O'Hare's voice-over description of the Californian location as if it were Iraq or Afghanistan adds to the contagion of differences that are normally kept separate, while the family's comedic exiting of their vehicle after the blast returns us to business as usual, i.e. the business of films to entertain, thereby preventing the viewer's satisfaction of a moral perspective on who is the victim, who is the perpetrator.

This frustration is exacerbated in the final sequence in which the real ex-drone operator's pixelated talking head briefly appears, his voice-over recounting his dawning realization that the laser targeting marker he operates via his computer at the Creech Air Force Base near Las Vegas, referred to by operators as 'the light of God', actually kills people. As he recounts this, the camera sweepingly revolves around the Stratosphere observation tower just off the Las Vegas strip. This building is a hotel and casino owned and operated by the gaming company Golden Entertainment. The camera speedily circles the tip of the tower and its gaudy lights, the nauseatingly smooth camera motion echoing the lack of physical repercussion in virtual, legally sanctioned killing, that is being prosaically described by the ex-operator.[16] The visual seduction of this scene of untrammelled movement through virtual space, in conjunction and disjunction with the story being recounted, paradoxically exacerbates the crime by uniting war and entertainment. It also performs a weird kind of realism that destabilizes moral certainty about where we are placed in relation to what we are seeing. The pharmacological nature of this sequence is that, rather than simply being a seductive accommodation to violence and trauma, it takes the viewer through a scenario that is unthinkable or intolerable in life, creating a homeopathic pathway through its sickness. What I mean here is that the sickness of an image technology that enables killing-at-a-distance is treated with images and sounds that, in their conflation of entertainment and trauma, are themselves sick by proxy. This is Shaviro's homeopathic magic, a form of homeopathic mimicry that treats like with like.

Accelerationist aesthetics

In *Post Cinematic Affect*, Shaviro claims that it is only film and video works which are fully immersed in the conditions of today's globalized network society that have the power to express the dangerous modulations of the neoliberal logic of perpetual crisis and catastrophe. We live in states of constant alert, subject to an existential anxiety that also finds traction in sociological literature such as that by Furedi and Illouz, both of whom refer to the transformation of trauma into generalized anxiety in neoliberal capitalism. Countering the mid-twentieth-century idea that art plays an oppositional role, which is deemed no longer plausible, Shaviro advances a strategy of 'homeopathic magic' in which film and artworks treat the sickness of neoliberal capitalist society by hyperbolically mimicking it. In this, films and videos that mirror the delirium of speculative finance and its overwhelming effects on the human sensorium are related to an accelerationist aesthetics. He derives this aesthetic from political accelerationism which according to Benjamin Noys aimed 'to exacerbate capitalism to the point of collapse' (Noys in Shaviro, 2010: 136). Shaviro quite rightly points out that this is a politically dubious idea as it does not offer any positive strategy of how the convulsive death of capitalism would lead to liberation rather than barbarism. However, Shaviro advocates it as an aesthetic strategy. This would entail the exacerbated performative mimicry of the sickening elements of capitalistic media culture, e.g. intense happenings as varied as explosions, weather fronts, criminal and sexually transgressive behaviour, in order to have them hit a rock bottom inefficacy, the exhausting of their possibilities resulting in a kind of affirmative negation. By following the trajectory of such characters or situations, Shaviro claims the viewer is effected at a deep visceral level such that they too become detached from belief in global capital's narrative of untrammelled regeneration and rampant competition. Not just this though. In showing us characters who survive in and beyond this climate, they also afford the hopeful vision that 'something needs to remain incommensurable, non-negotiable, unexchangeable outside the circle of capital' (Shaviro, 2010: 63).

While politically dubious, Shaviro's model, which I term 'homeopathic mimicry', is nonetheless a compelling way to approach gallery films such as Fast's. In the closing moments of *5000 Feet is the Best*, the camera eye floats from on high over the Las Vegas strip and the blocks of military suburban housing on the outskirts of the city, while the ex-drone operator describes what a potential human target looks like from 5000 feet: 'if someone gets up from sitting down they leave a heat cloud of white that looks like a flower to the surveillance eye.' To the ex-drone operator, the moment of the kill appears on-screen like a heavenly messenger, a 'quite beautiful' light. The equation of the killing machine to an angel accelerates the ex-drone pilot's sickness to a limit point in the film in which it implodes, quite literally, as the screen is illuminated by a whiting out similar to that which also occurs when the fireball erupts in *The Casting*. The moral implications of this implosion lie beyond the film, its job being to accompany us to that point, immersing us in a space in which we are contagiously effected by the sickness, but able to survive it unlike the populations living under constant threat of drones who have no means of psychic insulation.[17] Fast's immunizing inoculations are for Western audiences. His dissociative forms of storytelling creatively rework symptoms that do not master them but provide a homeopathic remedy for the poisonous knowledge that one is both culpable and powerless in relation to the macropolitical decisions taken by world leaders without the consent of the people they govern. The film's homeopathic impetus may be used by its audience like a transitional object that serves to immunize the subject so that they may tolerate or acknowledge poison without denying the pleasure of fabulation. Decades before Shaviro, Walter Benjamin suggested that film, in its use of percussive energies and haptic durations, might offer a buffer to the shock effects and threats of everyday life.[18] For Benjamin, the buffoon-like violence of Mickey Mouse was a kind of necessary, albeit nightmarish, immunization against the real violence of technification. Miriam Bratu Hansen cites Benjamin:

> If one considers the dangerous tensions which technification and its consequences have engendered [...] tendencies which at critical stages take on a psychotic character – one also has to recognize that this same technification has created the possibility of psychic immunization against such mass psychoses. It does so by means of certain films in which the forced development of sadistic fantasies and their masochistic delusions can prevent their natural and dangerous maturation in the masses. (in 2004: 29)

In 'Room-for-Play' (2004), Hansen makes the case that Benjamin was trying to posit film as a kind of play that, at the very least, might neutralize the damaging effects and uses of 'technification'. For me this is akin to how a technologized transitional space might function in providing the fabular film object that enables the viewer/infant to tolerate the imbrication of the toxic and the curative in a safely mediated environment. This is not a big leap to make given Benjamin's interest in Freudian psychoanalysis and his comparison of film to a publicly shared form of dreaming. To some extent, I am reading Fast's films as cinematic treatments that afford the gallery viewer a protective space, somewhat akin to Winnicott's transitional space of reality-testing, in which to explore the ramifications of toxicity without being damaged by it. Without this protection, a viewer, when confronted with the poisons of war and its traumatic aftermath, may either take a moral stance or find it emotionally overwhelming. Both these positions give satisfaction, the former of intellectual certainly, the latter of a reassuring empathy, neither of which unsettles our categories of good and evil. In a pharmacological aesthetics, these binaries are unsettled, the boundaries between reality and fantasy are held in abeyance while the infant/viewer undertakes a less censored imaginative exploration of them. However, unlike the emphasis on restorative wholeness advocated by many applications of Winnicott to the aesthetic field,[19] a pharmacological aesthetics enables remaining *with* the destabilization of boundaries as to do otherwise would be to use the artwork to deny the toxic pathologies of global capitalism.

As an aesthetics, what I call homeopathic mimicry immunizes us against the poisons that circulate in the system without eradicating them. While this is undoubtedly a privileged position by contrast to the states of anxiety suffered by those living under the constant threat of being vaporized by drone strikes, I want to end with an example of fieldwork that reinforces the necessity of aesthetic forms to surviving in the aftermath of traumatic experience. In December 2018, I participated in a panel on 'Anxiety, Health and Capitalism' at Ravensbourne University, organized by the Culture Capital Exchange, a company promoting the exchange of university partners' knowledge and expertise with business, cultural and creative sectors. One of the speakers, Dr Ayesha Ahmad, a global health lecturer, presented a research project she worked on at University College London to develop a therapeutic intervention for trauma using traditional storytelling for women who have experienced gender-based violence in extreme settings such as Afghanistan, Pakistan, Iran, Turkey and the Middle East. The project involved collaborating with staff running safe spaces for women suffering from the psychic effects of war crimes such as rape, their traumatizing experiences rendering them silent. Her approach in working, in this case, with Afghan women, was not to enlist them in therapeutic practices that might encourage them to speak their trauma, it being a Western notion that it is necessary to confess one's trauma in order to process and integrate it, an idea foreign to the cultures she was engaging with. Instead, in group workshops, she used the poetry that is part of the women's heritage. As forms of transgenerational expression, the poems often express sadness and loss, as well as pleasure. They are objects that can be used to presentify traumatic experience, not as something that has happened to me, but as a transpersonal transmission that operates between truth and fiction. Engaging with the poems enabled the silenced women to speak and to indirectly express their trauma as a transgenerational sharing beyond the individual self. A poem or a filmwork cannot prevent warfare but by creating a transitional space in which its traumas can be negotiated through imaginative projection, itself a kind of dissociation, it may re-channel their toxicity to create an immunization that preserves one's power to act elsewhere.

5

Melanie Gilligan's signifying semiologies and the micro-resistance of collective subjectivity

In the previous chapter, I discussed how media narratives might deploy a strategy of homeopathic mimicry, which, instead of offering counter-narratives to the psychopathologies of cognitive and global capitalism, hyperbolically performs their ills. I suggested that such performances in Fast's videos generated a kind of inoculation effect on the viewer, thereby enabling an immersion in catastrophes such as global warfare, killing-at-a-distance and the symptoms of PTSD that we prefer not to imagine or think about unless we are personally effected. In this chapter, I want to examine how an artist might use a mode of homeopathic mimicry to perform a pedagogical critique of the catastrophic subjectivities of cognitive capitalism whose lack of immunity towards the extraction of value from their affective and cognitive labour seems all-pervasive. Melanie Gilligan's speculative narratives in her web-based episodic dramas – *Crisis in the Credit System* (2008), *Popular Unrest* (2010) and *The Common Sense* (2014) – can be said to evince the nightmarish vision of cognitive capitalism as that which 'entangle[s] the mind's activity' in economic production (Berardi in De Boever and Neidich, 2013: 19). As I mentioned in the introduction, Berardi often uses the term 'cognitive capitalism' to refer to the contemporary state of capitalism in which there is a '[r]ise to prominence of the intellectual, semiotic and affective content of work and its product' (Genosko and Thoburn in Berardi, 2011: 4). However, his preferred term to describe post-Fordist modes of production, semiocapitalism, further intimates the reliance of this economy on 'the mind, language and creativity as its primary tools for the production of value' (Berardi, 2009: 21). Given that Gilligan's web series deploy a number of signifying semiologies from dramatized speech and gesture to digital graphics and data metrics, in what follows, I shall align her narratives with Berardi's analysis of semiotics in cognitive or semiocapitalism. Arguing that Berardi sets up a binary that becomes productively undone in Gilligan's work, I shall go on to explore her deployment of what, Berardi's friend and associate, the psychiatrist Felix Guattari[1] calls a 'mixed semiotics'. Rather than positing an alternative to cognitive capitalist capture, 'mixed semiotics' signals the possibility of micro-resistance within its parameters. This aesthetic involves going beyond homeopathic mimicry, but first I shall introduce how Gilligan's homeopathic treatment operates as a pedagogical tool.

Commenting on her pedagogical impetus, Gilligan says:

> when I started making my drama about the financial crisis, *Crisis in the Credit System*, I started to try to address what I thought was truly *needed* in the world. I made a work that was inserted into mass culture (without aping its forms or content) because I thought that the film was needed in that context, at that moment. [...] I began making the film with the idea that people needed to know about the financial crisis as the event would have a profound impact on all aspects of our increasingly financialized world. (in Donovan, 2012: online)

Although Gilligan here asserts that her work does not ape the forms and content of mass culture, *Crisis in the Credit System*,[2] a four-part web-based drama commissioned by Artangel Interaction specifically to be viewed online, nonetheless borrows media tropes of docu-drama and corporate video. The episodes track financial analysts who work for an investment banking firm as they participate in a role-playing seminar set in an Arcadian setting typical of corporate away days.[3] Echoing a group therapy workshop, the participants are instructed by the leader to improvise ways to cope with a volatile marketplace rather than with their own personal psychopathologies. The implication is that the market itself is sick, a condition the financial analysts are exhorted to remedy by coming up with imaginative solutions, which are presented as mini-narratives within the film.[4] Their ideas extracted, the workshop leader then announces their redundancy, implying that a new flexible workforce will take over the implementation of their ideas. By contrast to the analysts' desperation to perform successfully, one of the characters imagined by them in their role-playing exercises is a trader who, operating at the fictitious company

Delphi Capital Management, has a telepathic ability to intuit the turbulence of markets and to make investment forecasts on this affective basis. In being able to decode cognitive capitalism's recombinant logic of flux and flow, his sensibility corresponds with the financial graphics and metrics that are superimposed on his body. Moving to the beat of their algorithmic signals, he is the epitome of the info-worker in cognitive capitalism, as characterized by Berardi. 'Info-producers are neuro-workers. Their nervous systems act as active receiving terminals. They are sensitive to semiotic activation throughout the entire day' (Berardi, 2010: online). For Berardi this kind of semiotic activation, modelled as it is on electronic modes of communication, produces psychopathologies such as anxiety, depression and stress. In fact, Gilligan's fictitious trader eventually implodes from the informational overload that passes through his body, though there is a sense in the film that this kind of implosion is part and parcel of the cycle of creative destruction that enables capitalism to mutate and develop new markets as well as expanding the areas of life that can be subjected to financialization.[5] It is against the backdrop of this constant mutation that Berardi proposes withdrawal from the sphere of 'neuromobilization and constant creativity' in which the language of innovation and the production of new knowledge rule.

Connective semiocapitalism

Berardi characterizes the dominant semiotic model in cognitive or semiocapitalism as operating by means of connection rather than conjunction. In what he calls connective semiocapitalism, 'affects, attitudes, attributes and ideas [are] directly productive' (Genosko and Thoburn in Berardi, 2011: 5) rather than mediated through a triangulation of body, matter, machine or techne. Cognitive workers are involved in 'the elaboration of segments or "semiotic artefacts" that are highly abstract entities combined and recombined through an exploitative digital network only at the precise time they are required' (in Berardi, 2011: 5). Maintaining that the temporality of recombinant logic punctures the rhythms of human embodiment, Berardi states that:

> Multitasking implies the quick shift from an informational frame to another. The human mind seems to be perfectly suited to perform multitasking, but these kind of practices are triggering a psychological mutation, and this mutation is producing new forms of mental suffering like panic, attention deficit disorders, burnout, mental exhaustion, depression. (2014: 35)

As I shall describe further, in Gilligan's trilogy, characters' emotions and behaviours are interfaced by digital surveillance and quantification to such a degree that they seem to have no private or unconscious life. However, a paper co-authored with Marina Vishmidt offers a glimpse of how Gilligan's work might be seen as both diagnostic and remedial, a point I shall return to after discussing Berardi's connective semiocapitalism further. Gilligan and Vishmidt write that while

> [i]nvoluntary actions, reactions, and sensations are fed into the social reproduction of capital, yet the experience of the involuntary has no preformed relation to knowledge; *there is no image for what is happening.* The supposed irrationality of somatic and affective responses often obeys other nondiscursive rationalities, inscribing oppressions, subjugation, and even abstractions on a corporeal level. In this way, capital's formations are inscribed in social habit. Yet the gestures that result can fall anywhere on the political spectrum, in the service of the radical or the reactionary. (2018, my emphasis)

Berardi's approach to the 'radical' is to contrast the modular recombinatory logic of the technologies that underpin transactional life in cognitive capitalism to the language of conjunction, i.e. poetry, as that which unites images and ideas in metaphorical singularized meanings. As opposed to the connective time of digital communication that 'reduces different temporalities to a single measure' (Berardi, 2007), conjunction enables what Berardi refers to as a becoming other that singularizes the subject. He says that '[s]ingularities change when they conjoin, they become something other than what they were before their conjunction [whereas] connection entails a simple effect of machine functionality' (2007: online). For Berardi, semiocapitalism's 'insertion of the electronic in the organic, the proliferation of artificial devices in the organic universe, the body, communication and society' results in a transformation of the relationship between consciousness and sensibility in which 'the exchange of signs undergoes a process of an increasing desensitization' (Berardi, 2011: 40). In the face of this toxic cellularization of labour in cognitive capitalism, Berardi maintains that a language of conjunction needs to be preserved or revitalized.[6] In fact, Berardi goes so far as to link the language of conjunction, i.e. poetry, with therapy, stating that 'poetry and therapy (thera-poetry) will be the forces leading to the creation of a [...] cognitariat sensibility' (2011: 163) beyond political parties and the organizational interests of capital. To achieve this, he advocates the withdrawal of productivity from the cognitive capitalist sphere of 'neuromobilization and compulsory creativity' (2011: 36). Here he shows his Autonomist credentials which were aligned with 1960s and 1970s Italian Workerism, a movement that used the refusal to work, in conjunction with the wage struggle, as a resistance to the exploitative conditions of industrial capitalist production. However, contemporary forms of exploitative labour, both at the high-tech end of neuro-working and digital creativity and, at the other end of the scale, in the care and service economies (which I shall explore in Chapter 9), are not united by precarity and the struggle for wages. As Silvia Federici explains, Autonomist theories of precarious and immaterial labour only speak to the situation and interest of workers working at the highest level of capitalistic technology (2006). Although the electronic devices that organize transactional life in cognitive capitalism serve to connect people across the globalized world of dispersed labour and displacement (due to war and poverty), it is also the case that in highly technologized environments, such devices exacerbate voluntary subjection to their electronic pulse. For Berardi, this results in a 'becoming sensitive to the code, to sudden changes of state, and to the sequence of discrete signs' (2011: 40). He calls this a 'desensitization of the sinuous' (2011: 40). For him, these machinic rhythms lack the ambiguity and semantic interpretation of the poetic mode of conjunction. However, Berardi's contrast between connection and conjunction in which the latter is viewed as a semiotic resistance to the colonization of human experience in the former is not consistently maintained in his writing. In 'Sensitivity to the Rhizome' (2007), he puts forward a more ambivalent vision of 'posthuman transition [that] revolves around the alternative between conjunction and connection and takes the realm of sensibility as its main object [...] sensibility to change, departure, flow and beauty' (2007, online). This suggests that the disentanglement of sensibility from the disruptive pulse of connectivity that he often calls for can also entail working with these rhythms rather than rejecting them tout court. Something of this working with and against the disruptive yet all-pervasive pulse of connectivity emerges in Gilligan's 'trilogy', her fictions both presenting an exacerbation of this condition of subjection and a reimagining of its potential for subjectivation, i.e. the production of new forms of autonomous subjectivity.

Gilligan's collective subjectivities

Much as Fast's multivalent narrative structures divorced the symptoms of PTSD from individual pathology, Gilligan is also interested in separating emotions from particular characters, instead creating emotional assemblages in which characters participate in collective feelings. Discussing her intentions for *Popular Unrest*, a fictional docu-drama in five episodes that straddles the genres of horror and sci-fi, she says:

> When I made *Popular Unrest* [...] I opened up a Pandora's Box by experimenting in creating non-individual subjects – i.e. I developed that film using acting workshops in which I asked the group of actors to work together to make up different aspects of a particular person or of an emotional state. I was trying to push for a *breakdown* of individual, separate characters and to see if I could depart from making the type of drama that is premised on this separation. (Gilligan in Donovan, 2012, italics mine)

As well as being presented online, *Popular Unrest* is also shown in galleries on five separate monitors in booths formed by office screens and plastic dividers, an installation format that echoes the kinds of corporate spaces portrayed in the film. In the gallery, the episodes follow on one from the other, although, given that some are slightly longer than others, the viewer occasionally enters some way into an episode, a factor which mirrors televisual viewing in domestic space. Like any of the cult dramas such as *CSI* and *Dexter*, which provide some inspiration for *Popular Unrest*, the episodes conclude with a cliff-hanger that incites anticipation for the next instalment, and akin to the streaming platforms that characterize TV viewing in a digital age, one doesn't have to wait until the following week to find out what happens next. Although there are many DIY aspects to the film, for example the blood spatter bags, the work's production values mimic those of advertising and TV news, it being possible to do this on a relatively low budget due to current developments of digital technology.

Popular Unrest explores whether there is any aspect of human life and social interaction which escapes the technological and disciplinary systems of capture characteristic of late or cognitive capitalism. The film is set in a future similar to now except that paper has been done away with and the incursion into *bios* by capital, i.e. the governance of populations' life worlds, has happened to such a degree that all emotional needs and desires are measured and evaluated by computerized systems that feed into an overarching organism called 'the Spirit', a metaphor for capitalism in the film that draws on Karl Marx's critique of Hegel. People are seen going about their daily routines in a clinical, cool manner: working out in gyms; at work in banks and call centres; all activities contributing to Big Data's monitoring of their bodily weight, energies and sleep patterns for future predictions. Gilligan says: '*Popular Unrest* looks at how capital manages and captures the future behavior and physical health of populations' (Gilligan in Holert, 2012: 87). However, this efficiency is being disrupted by random murders, though no killer appears in the episodes, just a knife stabbing the sacks of blood-like liquid. Seemingly, the logic of 'the Spirit' is that once it has reached a certain level of glut, it is necessary to eradicate some 'data', transforming it into the raw meat underlying the cognitive capitalist concept of the body as an agglomeration of neural transmitters that can be regulated under the right scientific conditions. As Gilligan says: 'Throughout *Popular Unrest*, there are many satirical renderings of the ways that the private and public sphere today turn one's choices regarding one's physical and financial "health" into a permanent state of social liability' (Gilligan in Holert, 2012: 89). For me, this aspect of the narrative relates to how capitalist production and biopolitical governance depend on the eradication or genocide of some global populations, though the series keeps it local and light-hearted.

The main actors in the film are introduced to us via a documentary voice-over as being 'a good representative cross section of London's urban population', who have been telepathically drawn to an abandoned warehouse. The members of the group feel a strong empathetic connection to one another that they explore further using team bonding exercises and role-play. Their enactments of emotional trauma emerge out of a seemingly benign desire for connection with one another, but this is precisely how 'the Spirit', i.e. capital, infiltrates their bodies at the neurological level. In one of the most compelling episodes, the group members, wired up to a data collecting machine, are being observed from behind glass by a team of scientists while they perform remembered gestures and behaviours that replicate acts of labour and work. As their movements are measured, they are translated into neuro-physiological data monitored by scientists on behalf of 'the Spirit'. The visual metrics of this data intermittently appear superimposed on or constraining group members' bodies, their gestures gaining in speed in conjunction to the beat of the fast-paced electronic soundtrack. The scene could be said to echo Berardi's description of cognitive capitalism which 'puts neuro-psychic energies to work, submitting them to mechanistic speed, compelling cognitive activity to follow the rhythm of networked productivity. As a result, the emotional sphere linked with cognition is stressed to its limit' (2010).

Popular Unrest acutely diagnoses how 'an instrumental logic of exchange and profit' (Gilligan in Holert 89) subjects cognitive workers to precarious autonomous conditions that generate the psychopathologies that Berardi, Stiegler, Han and others have identified, e.g. depression and anxiety, panic and fear: the former being considered a drain on the economy, while the

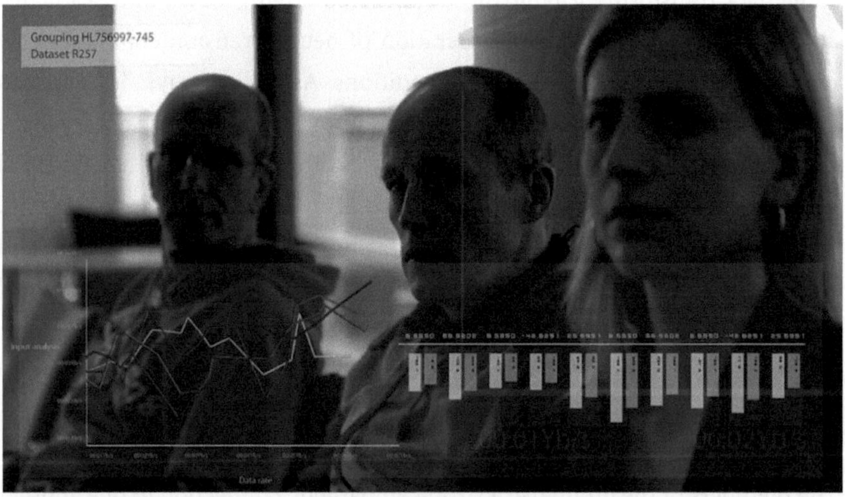

Figure 5.1 Melanie Gilligan, *Popular Unrest*, 2010; Courtesy the artist and Galerie Max Mayer, Düsseldorf.

latter two propagate the competitive spirit that drives it (Davies, 2015). In the episode I've just described, bodies are shown breaking down and burning out, symptoms that litter the contemporary psychosphere. The biopolitical processes of what I am referring to as cognitive capitalism create both self-regulating and vulnerable subjects who require therapeutic aid to function in its precarious sites of work and education. Yet the seeking out of therapeutic aid to bolster the self reproduces the vulnerability that prompts the seeking of help in the first place. To supposedly offset this individual cycle of risk and vulnerability, many Western corporations and establishments embed team bonding exercises and activities as almost mandatory. Yet, this care for the employee is fully bound up with the logic of production. As Illouz has documented, the language of therapy pervaded management culture since the 1970s when old-style factory labour and its ethos of keeping control of one's emotions shift to the notion that expressing one's emotions at work is a way of increasing productivity (Illouz, 2007). While emotional sharing, role-playing and the improvisational working through of problems may generate a sense of camaraderie, they are ultimately for the sake of producing more 'info-capital' or 'neuro-work' for corporations who benefit economically from this mode of surplus value. In fact, Gilligan's film suggests that this very capacity to feel one another's feelings, to empathize with one another, is the channel by which capital can enter their bodies so as to extract more surplus value from areas of life that were previously thought to be external to capitalist valorization processes. As Sven Lütticken says: 'In the post-Fordist economy, as service jobs become more important, it became imperative to present oneself not so much as an interchangeable supplier of labor-power [...] but to perform oneself as a unique commodity-person' (2005: 17). But the paradox, as gleaned from the range of gestures performed by Gilligan's group, is that in this society of performative subjects, 'the actors – we, potentially everyone – are assemblages, montages of repetitions' with the result that 'citation has to operate within narrow limits, without much variation' (Lütticken, 2005: 19).

Instead of using their telepathic powers to become a force to be reckoned with, Gilligan's group members willingly deliver themselves up to having their affective neuro-mobilizations studied to further contribute to the workings of 'the Spirit'. And their search to track down this abstract entity, which initially seemed to suggest a desire for resistance, ends up in the final episode with them joining with 'the Spirit' in a stabbing frenzy that they survive in 'Spirit' heaven, safe from the effects of violent protests by populations across the globe. Pixelated mobile phone footage from the then recent revolts across the Arab Spring countries appear on the screen, as the voice-over describes how these riots generated even more inequalities of distribution. Those who could afford it built gated communities sealed off from the violence, capitalism speedily recovering from the destructive force of the protests, epitomizing economist Joseph Schumpeter's diagnosis that capitalism operates by means of creative destruction.[7] Recalling my citation above of Gilligan's and Vishmidt's paper, it could be said that Gilligan's narrative flounders in trying to provide an 'image' that might show how 'the involuntary' (here figured as protest) need not be corralled as reactionary. As she ruminates:

> People seemed battered by decades of neoliberal attack. For this reason, so many things that happen with the groupings in the film are representations of obstacles to social solidarity today: the way the groupings interpret their mysterious feeling of connectedness as having subjective or emotional cause, thinking it is either an emotional understanding borne out of distress and hard times [. . .], or perhaps even a psychic connection. (in Holert, 2012: 92)

Unlike Shaviro's identification of homeopathic mimicry in media narratives in which the implosion of the catastrophic subjectivities of capitalism, as represented by the characters, preserves something outside the sphere of commodification, Gilligan's diagnostic vision is cruelly dystopian.[8] In fact, Gilligan's critique of Catherine Sullivan's six-screen video installation *The Chittendens* (2005) could equally be applied to her own work. For Gilligan, *The Chittendens* did not open up a political dimension but simply offered 'the spectacular mirror image of a post-Fordist demand for frequent and surplus transformation' (2007: 430). Her view of the often skittish gestures performed by Sullivan's sixteen performers dressed in costumes based on stereotypes in nineteenth- and twentieth-century America – the Secretary, the Muscle Man or the Management Executive – is that they mirror Paolo Virno's theorization of virtuosity in which the performative, communicative aspect of contemporary labour renders politics another branch of performance. By contrast, Gilligan's intention is to wake spectators up from this spell by creating an image of 'the total social capital' so that viewers might see that 'the Spirit is not the totality but that we are and that capital's mediation of our actions both unites and puts all our activity into abstract relation' (in Holert, 2012: 88). But, as J. Jasper Bernes states, and I somewhat agree:

> One might be tempted to interpret *Popular Unrest* as a ruthlessly functionalist account of capital, not to mention a politically pessimistic one, a one-sided dialectic in which capital always gets what capital needs. Such a view is also implicit in the account of crisis given in *Crisis in the Credit System*, where breakdown is regenerative, a form of creative destruction, and part of capitalism's overcoming of its own barriers. (Bernes, 2015)

However, might there be another way of considering what an image of the involuntary would look like or how it might operate in Gilligan's diagnostic narratives?

Guattari's signifying semiotics

To enable me to think through this counterintuitive idea, I shall first turn to Berardi's colleague Guattari, not only because of his claims that the semiotic operator of what he calls Integrated World Capitalism provides the tools of resistance within itself, but also because of his vested interest and career in the psychotherapeutic profession.[9] While Guattari has written specifically on aesthetics in *Chaosmosis: An Ethico-Aesthetic Paradigm* (1995), here I want to look at some earlier texts that focus on semiosis and on cinema, both of which allow me to address Gilligan's work in terms of how the pharmacology of using mainstream media forms might re-canalize (Stiegler's term for re-channel) subjectivity.

Rather than the predominant opposition between connection and conjunction in Berardi's semiotics, Guattari suggests that the 'a-signifying semiotics' of electronic signals and code (i.e. connection) might offer the potential in aesthetic practices for 'another organization of reality' (Guattari in Seem, 1974: 39), one that might bypass dominant power agendas. Guattari's theory of expression is propped on three different classifications of signifying systems or what he also calls 'encodages', a French term for the production of meaning by means of a code and that remains untranslated in the interview I am referring to here (Guattari in Seem, 1974: 39). Firstly, there are 'the a-semiotic encodages, these being all the "natural" codings' such as genetic codings for example' (1974: 39). (This is reminiscent of the genome in Stiegler's first order of memory and will not concern my analysis here.) Secondly, he adumbrates what he calls 'semiological encodages'. These comprise two elements: on the one hand, the signifying semiologies of language, i.e. signifiers and signifieds and the laws that govern their usage. But also the presignifying semiologies which 'function at the level, for example, of primitive societies, of childhood, of madness etc. [...] For example, a substance of (gestural) expression, of verbal expression, of inscriptions on the body, of dance, of posture systems, etc.' (Guattari in Seem, 1974: 39). In considering these 'presignifying semiologies', which are the terrain of aesthetic practices, on a semiotic continuum with 'signifying semiologies', Guattari not only departs from Saussurean-inspired theories of signification, but also puts a dampener on the idea that artistic expressions and forms intrinsically challenge the status quo, as many artists and art educators maintain. However, Guattari also proposes a third order comprising code and electronic signals that he sees as having some potential to resist capture, what he calls 'a-signifying semiotics, sign machines which operate independently of any and all production of meaning' (1974: 39). This claim is hard to take on board given the current enmeshment of Big Data with biopolitical governance. However, his allusion to the micro-political value of what he calls '*mixed semiotics*, semiotics which participate in both systems - a-signifying semiotics, and signifying semiologies' (Guattari in Seem, 1974: 40, emphasis original) seems more conducive to my purposes in analysing Gilligan's pharmacological aesthetics. Describing the mixed semiotics of audio-visual systems such as cinema and television, Guattari says that:

> there is an overlapping of the semiotic of the image, a semiology of speech, a semiology of sounds, of noises, semiotics of corporeal expression and then, on another side, these mixed semiotics are also signifying semiologies. That is to say that Power, the many different power systems, pull all these towards the side of a semiology of the dominant values, whereas they tend to function, from the point of view of their own constitution, as semiotics of desire. (1974: 40)

The upshot of this for artistic practices is the potential of a mixed semiotics in dissociating sensation and affect, i.e. the sensibility, from the economic regime of exchange value. This does not mean that the sensibility will not be captured by dominant power systems, but that, as Gilligan and Vishmidt propose, the gestures that result from affective and somatic responses 'can fall anywhere on the political spectrum, in the service of the radical or the reactionary' (2018). While I think Guattari is overly optimistic about the neutrality of 'a-signifying semiotics', there may be a case to be made that as part of a 'mixed semiotics', they might produce a sensibility that cannot be fully captured by dominant power. For Guattari, while 'machines of mixed semiotics, such as television, cinema etc., capture the desires of the masses and put these to the uses of the signifying machines of Authority' (in Seem, 1974: 40), they also have the potential to delink desire from the latter due the unconscious production of 'a-signifying semiotics' that operate in tandem to coded signification. The productive force of 'a-signifying semiotics' operate by means of what Guattari calls a machinic unconscious which is unlike the Freudian one of repression.[10] The notion of a machinic unconscious might seem less strange if we think of the associational processes of the dream work as itself a machine, an analogy that Guattari makes in *Anti-Oedipus: Capitalism and Schizophrenia* (2000 [1972]) which he co-authored with Gilles Deleuze. Rather than simply being opposed to psychoanalysis, they appropriate the Freudian unconscious as a machine whose cogs and wheels are forever accumulating and generating new material configurations that they call assemblages. These assemblages often repeat dominant identitarian structures but they also channel the potential of desire beyond the control of consciousness. According to Guattari:

> At any and every level, on the large or the small scales, a revolutionary micro-politics of the libido might exist, a type of system of escape or evasion which places different orders in connection, as well as different semiotics: but there can also always be a recovery, a totalitarian politics of the libido which can, basically, characterize the paranoiac economy, itself part of a molar organization. In other words, the struggle, as we have never stopped saying, is not situated in a privileged way at one particular level. (in Seem, 1974: 40)

This is not to say that 'a-signifying semiotics' are radical in themselves but that in their proximity to the irrational 'encodages' of the psyche, they may, in conjunction with dominant forms of signification, produce a new kind of subjectivity that partially evades capture.

This idea is further underscored in Guattari's two short essays on cinema in *Chaosophy* (2009), both of which are relevant to my argument here. In his essay 'Cinema of Desire', Guattari writes that while cinema's technological development subjected the immediate intensities of silent film to the dominance of discursive narrative, the cinema machine still carries traces of these intensities that (unpredictably) resound and reverberate through the grid of signifying semiologies (language, stories, discourse). And in 'The Poor Man's Couch', he suggests that this may be the case because 'the semiotic components of film glide by each other without fixing or stabilising' (2009: 263). As a machine of 'mixed semiotics', film's a-signifying and signifying components, while being organized by dominant Power, are not fully controlled by it.

However, Guattari can afford to be optimistic given that the audio-visual codes of technology at his time of writing, i.e. television, cinema and the early internet, appeared to have less of a biopolitical stronghold on psychic desire. By contrast, Berardi is witness to the oppressive form of Big Data, its racist and sexist biases, as well as how dominant power interests are being served by high-tech companies such as Google, Facebook and PayPal which have extended reach into the biopolitical governance of contemporary life.[11] However, the potential of Guattari's 'mixed semiotics' has been updated by philosopher Maurizio Lazzarato in a way that bears on my interpretation of Gilligan's *The Common Sense*. Before going on to look at this last film in what could loosely be called a trilogy, I want to briefly elaborate Lazzarato's expansion of Guattari's theory of semiotics in the context of cognitive capitalism.[12]

Updating Guattari's 'a-signifying semiotics' for a post-internet generation, Lazzarato's thesis is that subjectivity is produced at the point of intersection between 'social subjection and machinic enslavement' (2014a: 13–14). Lazzarato aims to understand how machines of mixed semiotics, although operating to control and capture psychological desire, are also productive of resistance. Following Guattari, he proffers 'the cinema machine' as an apparatus for subjection and enslavement, but equally, its a-signifying semiotics 'can also be turned into new processes for subjectivation provided that one recognize the nature of machinic assemblages' (Lazzarato, 2014a: 138). (Note that subjectivation relates to the production of subjectivity, whereas subjection has to do with being subject to oppression.) In order to construct a politics beyond what Lazzarato views as the pathologies of cognitive capitalism, i.e. beyond exploitation, racism, war and colonialism, all of which centre on the human, he advocates the necessity of both taking advantage of and acting against the deterritorialization of meaning put in play by the 'a-signifying semiotics' of algorithms and data (2014a). Lazzarato's list of 'a-signifying semiotics' includes data, algorithms, stock listings, currencies and equations. Something of both acting with and against the deterritorialization effected by a-signifying semiotics could be said to be played out in the machinic assemblages in Gilligan's *Popular Unrest*, although acting against their deterritorialization is overly prescriptive in her literal image of protest. More radical might be her assemblage of all three of Guattari's signifying semiologies without being subsumed by any of them, so that something might 'slip past' (Lazzarato, 2014a: 80). While her homeopathic mimicry of life under cognitive capitalism clearly resonates with Stiegler's aforementioned, 'Phew! [...] It's out. Our illness has been articulated' (2014: 41), Gilligan's assembly of characters in conjunction with the different registers of signifying semiologies at play in her films gestures towards the unpredictability of desire and imagining otherwise.

Feeling that she did not go far enough in *Popular Unrest* in 'push[ing] for a breakdown of individual, separate characters' (in Donavan, 2012), Gilligan's next series *The Common Sense* features a vast number of characters who directly feed into one another's thoughts, sensations and feelings via a transmission device called 'The Patch'. The brilliance of this virtual interface is that it epitomizes the eradication of a medium that Berardi claims is a characteristic of connective communication. Worn by users on the roof of the mouth, this 'neural entrainment device' connects students to corporations and workers to employers in a neurological immediacy that erases the distinction between input and output, at least for those on the lower echelons of the service industries. The device is a means of harnessing emotional data to enhance productivity and eradicate unnecessary jobs, though at the same time, akin to Guattari's machines of 'mixed semiotics', it harbours the potential for a collective sharing of feelings and needs that Gilligan proposes might bypass capitalist economies of exchange. Gilligan describes the film:

> Conceptions such as empathy and solidarity have been replaced with the ability to have concrete sensations of other people's situations. [...] Collective political resistance is emerging in many places around the world. However, the technology's role in these shifts is ambiguous. There are just as many ways that the technology is useful to the needs of capital as there are ways that it creates new means of its overcoming. While this technological development creates possibilities for new modes of existence and collective social formations, it also leads to new contradictions and conflicts.[13]

Unlike the previous series', *The Common Sense* is not available online.[14] It currently exists as a multi-screen gallery installation comprising fifteen episodes in total, though it has been exhibited in multiples of five and ten. The episodes are displayed on individual monitors suspended at different angles on a metal modular frame that is configured across the space. There are a number of narrative strands in this speculative fiction, not all of which I shall go into here, as my purpose is to explore the potential of a 'mixed semiotics' to *image* involuntary sensibility beyond the purview of capital.

The fifteen episodes are divided into three Phases: Phase 1 and Phases 2A and 2B, each phase comprising five episodes of approximately six minutes each. Importantly, in the installation, the viewer's headset tunes in and out of the episodes as they come within range of each screen's sweet spot, thereby adding a sonic interference to the image stream that also partakes of the 'a-signifying semiotics' of the machinic as defined by Guattari. Shot mostly in the Netherlands, with some footage shot in Toronto, Phase 1 opens on a classroom in the Netherlands in which students watch a video about 'The Patch' as it existed ten years prior, the implication being that the students live in a future in which the technology is further developed. In fact, while watching the video history of 'The Patch', the students receive transmissions from their employers and information on their finances through the very latest 'patch' technology. After the screening, Gibson, the teacher, says: 'Of course, "The Patch" did make life a lot more collective, just not the way they expected. Their belief that being connected would mean that people would join together to fight for a better collective situation was false'. Her opening statement is a dystopian forewarning that Gilligan's investment in the potential of collective subjectivity has already failed. And certainly, it is clear from the first five episodes of Phase 1 that 'The Patch' has created more opportunities for monitoring the precarious labour force, including students, factory workers and service industry employees, to achieve maximal productivity. Akin to Shaviro's notion of the accelerative nature of homeopathic mimicry in media narratives, Phase 1 ends with a breakdown of 'The Patch' and an ensuing implosion. Given the students' immersion in the technology, the shock of its abandonment generates rampant hysteria before they collapse dejected in a dormitory-like space. After this, the narrative bifurcates into two strands, Phases 2A and 2B, the modular frame branching out in opposite directions like a T-bar,[15] which, for the gallery viewer, means making a choice about which strand to follow. Both Phases deploy a 'mixed semiotics' of shot documentary and staged footage, cell and software animation, mobile phone footage and news media reportage of actual protests in 2011 and 2012, advertising graphics and data metrics as well as an electronic soundtrack that is interrupted by the crackling sound accompanying the movement of zoning in and out of the sweet spot. However, they diverge in their recounting of what happened after the breakdown of 'The Patch'.

Phase 2A mainly explores how people began to reduce their dependence on 'The Patch', exploring other types of 'technics' – books for example – and other types of collective solidarity such as protest movements. This is ostensibly the utopian side of the fiction. Phase 2B explores the more corporate development of the device and how it can be enhanced to produce even more interconnected empathic and entrained subjects with the aim of increasing profits for its investor, the venture capitalist, Liam. However, each of the bifurcating strands contains moments that do not adhere to the sharp distinction between good and bad uses of the technology, but pose contradictions that oscillate between being pharmacologically open-ended and frustratingly didactic, given that the installation's structural bifurcation had implied that there may be an alternative to the neural entrainment of workers in the cognitive capitalist economy.

In the previous chapter, I discussed Shaviro's idea that works of art that show the complete commodification of emotional experience act like a therapeutic dose of reality, not only in allowing us to acknowledge the encroachment of capital into areas of life that were once held apart from it, but also in giving us hope we can survive this incursion and the implosions it triggers. The assembly of characters in Phase 2A survives the implosion of 'The Patch' by testing

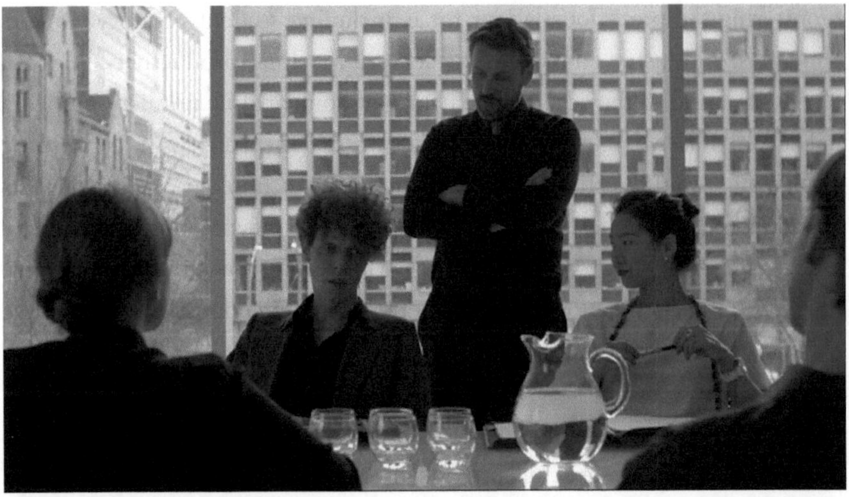

Figure 5.2 Melanie Gilligan, *The Common Sense*, 2014; Courtesy the artist and Galerie Max Mayer, Düsseldorf.

out different kinds of collectivities – protest marches, communal pedagogy for children, as well as, in the final episode of that strand, a self-organizing revolutionary group of eco-warriors dressed in camouflage gear. In Phase 2B's more dystopian strand, there are breakdowns of a different kind. This strand ends with a sequence of Liam, the venture capitalist, going AWOL, as if his megalomaniac fantasy of extracting fathomless profit from the neurological receptivity between people via 'The Patch' becomes the cause of his own unravelling. However, an implosion of a different order also occurs in the same episode. A fast-paced montage links shots of Victoria, the management info-worker in Phase 1, who uses 'The Patch' to receive transmissions from her surrogate's womb, with shots of her surrogate, Jackie, who works as a cleaner in the factory, and images of the foetus in her womb, as well as images of the factory machines, the speed of which increases in sync with the throbbing electronic soundtrack. The montage of shots of the two women seemingly choking to death in two different spaces is rapidly intercut, while the close-up shot of a foetal creature, filtered to look extremely alien, is statically held. Is this human embryo the new organ that researchers hope 'The Patch' will become or is it a potential for existential singularity in the wake of catastrophic implosion? The glowing luminosity of its red and orange 'intrauterine' fluid contrasts with the dirty greys in the complementary end scene of Phase 2A in which the group of post-apocalyptic eco-warriors assemble for a meeting. Might there be a possible connection between these two forms of potentiality both of which are poised on the brink of becoming something new without substantializing what this new production of subjectivity might be? Although I am reluctant to add another philosopher to the mix, Gilligan's allegory suggests to my mind a connection between Guattari's notion of how a 'mixed semiotics' carries signifying elements that bypass codification and Hannah Arendt's notion of 'natality'.

Wolfhart Totschnig explains that for Arendt 'natality (i.e. our condition of being born) is the "source" or "root" of our capacity to begin (i.e. of our capacity to initiate something new)' (2017: 329). Clarifying that Arendt does not mean birth as biological necessity but rather 'the arrival of newcomers in the web of human relations' (342), he posits this 'capacity to begin' as the basis of political action. In birth as natality, the uniqueness of the newcomer's life will not only elicit unpredictable responses from others, but also act towards others in unforeseen ways. For me, a resonant element of unpredictability emerges in the implosive exchange of transmissions between the two women and the foetal creature. Not only do we not know who will survive what seems to be a malfunction of 'The Patch', but there is also a sense that 'the newcomer' signifies the new sets of relations and actions that might come into being in a future beyond the work, a potentiality reminiscent of the hope characterized by Shaviro as remaining partly outside of exchange relations. On the other hand, however, rather than engendering 'new vectors of subjectivity', Gilligan's allegory seems to come down on what Guattari refers to as 'the individual as a terminal for data-processing machines' (Guattari 2000: 23). The collective protesters that assemble at the end of Phase 2A seem to be suspended in a liminal space without a purpose and one could also easily read the image of the foetal creature as a further incursion of capital into the life world of reproduction. However, the intense colour saturation and mute gesticulation in this relatively still, non-discursive shot could also be said to function as a more poetic image than the didactic narrative of the work as a whole. In other words, it acts more on the side of 'a-signifying semiotics'. While Gilligan predominantly forecloses on the unpredictability of life worlds within her urban techno-futures, the sound-image of 'natality' opens onto the unpredictability of future relations and actions. In intimating this, the work performs a pharmacological aesthetics that promises new modes of survival in full cognizance of the risks of poisonous transmission. This is admittedly a small glimpse of hope but its derivation from the 'a-signifying semiotics' of a sound-image that pivots on the brink of implosion without caving-in, gestures towards 'the radical'.

6

Pharmacological reparation in Liz Magic Laser's *Primal Speech*

In the previous chapter, I looked at Melanie Gilligan's speculative fictions in which characters implode under the pressure of connective cognitive capitalism's incursion into everyday life. Exploring the pharmacological aesthetic of her mimicry of this incursion, I deployed both Berardi's and Guattari's notions of semiotics, as well as Shaviro's notion of homeopathic magic, to raise the question of what might 'slip past' cognitive codification. In this chapter, I want to continue with this thematic in relation to Liz Magic Laser's installation *Primal Speech* (2016) whose film component is a fictional, documentary-style enactment loosely based on primal scream therapy. I shall argue that her deployment of this and other therapeutic discourses in this work oscillates between the two poles of the pharmakon as a poison (in its mimicry and critique of dominant power values) and a remedy (in its engendering of momentary respite and imaginative potential). Before I go on to look at Laser's work, I firstly want to introduce another aspect of Shaviro's pharmacological aesthetics which is connected to his notion of homeopathic magic. The purpose of this is to further establish a theoretical scene of critique that will progressively become undone in my encounter with *Primal Speech* towards the end of this chapter.

Shaviro's fear of breakdown

Shaviro's notion of homeopathic magic as a hyperbolic mimicry of the worst aspects of control society in which 'capital predicts, controls, and stockpiles the future [...] through a process of continual modulation' (Shaviro, 2010: 32) is an appropriation and development of Benjamin Noys' notion of political accelerationism, i.e. the exacerbation of capitalism to the point of collapse.[1] Shaviro's claim is that while accelerationism has been shown to be a dubious political strategy, it has value as an aesthetics in that, by mapping the toxic terrain of global capitalism through mimicry of it, it affords the prospect of generating affects and imagining futures not predicted by industry (Shaviro, 2010). I referred to this in the previous chapter. However, in his later *No Speed Limit* (2015), Shaviro further considers aesthetic accelerationism as an artistic strategy of 'aesthetic inefficacy', stating that:

> Aesthetic accelerationism does not even deny that its own intensities serve the aim of extracting surplus value and accumulating profit. The evident complicity and bad faith of these works, their reveling in the base passions that Nietzsche disdained, and their refusal to sustain outrage or claim the moral high ground: all these postures help to move us toward the disinterest and epiphenomenality of the aesthetic. So I don't make any political claims for this sort of accelerationist art [...] But I do want to claim a certain *aesthetic inefficacy* for them—which is something that works of transgression and negativity cannot hope to attain today. (Shaviro, 2015: 39–40, emphasis in original)

Rather than the kind of relationality inherent in Illouz' notion of immanent critique in which actors' desires are not simply conflictual, but only emerge from within the situations in which they are entangled (my sympathies lie here), Shaviro moves towards the Kantian notion of the aesthetic as disinterestedness. While this is not the direction of my argument, I want to remain with Shaviro's affirmative cynicism for the moment as it facilitates a way into the pharmacological aesthetics of Laser's *Primal Speech*, as well as retrospectively relating to the implosions that I identified in Gilligan's narratives.

Shaviro defines accelerationism as

> the argument that the only way out is the way through. In order to overcome globalized neoliberal capitalism, we need to drain it to the dregs, push it to its most extreme point, follow it into its furthest and strangest consequences. (2015: 2)

He further qualifies this by saying that '[i]ntensifying the horrors of contemporary capitalism does not lead them to explode, but it does offer us a kind of satisfaction and relief, by telling us that we have finally hit bottom, finally realized the worst' (2015: 35). For Shaviro, this realization is homeopathically curative in that it acknowledges the toxic reality of the situation and treats it according to the principle of like with like, i.e. the addition, through mimicry, of more toxicity. His cynical realism paradoxically finds an unlikely resonance with D.W. Winnicott's 'Fear of Breakdown' (1974), a paper that infers a more pharmacological approach to psychic development than the oftentimes benign register of Winnicott's transitional phenomena. In 'Fear of Breakdown', Winnicott discusses how, for patients whose psychic organization is spent warding off a fear of breakdown in the future, the realization that it has already happened in the past can be a way forwards. Relieved of channelling their psychic energies in search of a catastrophe they believed to be in the future, they can psychically reorient those energies towards present conditions. However, the realization that the worst has already happened has an ambivalent therapeutic edge to it. On the one hand, it breaks down the paranoid defensive mechanisms invented and rigidly adhered to by the ego to ward off future catastrophe, but, on the other hand, it releases the now vulnerable ego into a precarious state of being that necessitates the creation of new ways of moving forwards, a much more difficult trajectory. Loosely mapping this onto Shaviro's aesthetic theory and to the relation between a media work and its viewer or receiver, it could be said that media works that show us that 'the worst' has already happened might momentarily release the psychic energy that is otherwise spent constructing defence mechanisms against the fantasy of future breakdown. The projection of an aesthetic image of breakdown, witnessed in a public setting such as an art gallery, removes the fantasy from being an internalized psychopathology. In recognizing that 'the worst' has already happened, the 'bulldozer' concepts of neoliberalism and/or cognitive capitalism might seem minutely less incapacitating and so enable productive ways of working both with and against them. Although I do not revert to Shaviro's more Kantian notion of 'aesthetic inefficacy', nonetheless his idea that there is satisfaction in realizing that the worst has already happened, refracted through Winnicott's 'Fear of Breakdown', provides a context for my discussion of *Primal Speech*, a video installation in which 'the worst' as both psychic and social breakdown is hyperbolically performed, at least for a certain sector of people at the creative or high-tech end of Berardi's cognitariat. I explore how the exposure of this breakdown might enable and/or preclude the reparative side of the pharmacological, which is not about total healing but about being able to access the 'nourishing pleasures' (Buck-Morss in Kester, 1997: 45) of a transitional space in which toxicity might be assimilated without being eradicated or denied.

Therapeutic emotional style in Laser's work

Prior to *Primal Speech*, Laser explored the emotional, rhetorical style of speech-making that has taken over the public media and political spheres in performance media works such as *I Feel Your Pain* (2011), *The Digital Face* (2012), *Stand Behind Me* (2013) and *The Thought Leader* (2015). While her analysis in these works is inspired by the ideas of François Delsarte, who developed oratorical theories and exercises in the early nineteenth century, I would say that the tenor of the gestures and rhetorical content of her remediation of political speeches effect a decidedly therapeutic emotional style. In this, they tally with Furedi's diagnosis of how, from the 1970s onwards, politicians in both the United Kingdom and the United States began to be trained in such a style to engage and persuade the public by a blatant, yet persuasive, use of 'personal' feelings. He describes this as 'the ascendancy of therapeutic politics' which sets out to remedy a perceived social disengagement with conventional politics, a mistrust of authority and a growing alienation from the electoral system (2004: 45). In conjunction with this, and again of relevance to Laser's work, he states that 'increasingly news reporters want to know how a politician feels rather than what he or she has done' (2004: 44). Furedi gives the example of Bill Clinton telling the world about personal growth stories early in his presidency (58), as well as his later 'personal' apology to the nation for moral misconduct which, like all such numerous displays by politicians, attempt to garner pity by transmitting the message that 'like you, I feel pain' or, to riff on the parodic title of Laser's performance and moving image work: 'I feel *your* pain.' Such techniques pacify anger by making the populace feel that politicians are vulnerable too. By proffering the illusion that we are all equally in this together, biopolitical governance uses a therapeutic emotional style as a means of subjection.

Laser's *I Feel Your Pain* is a four-act play consisting of fourteen scenes which are enacted and filmed from within the audience and projected live on-screen.[2] The script comprises appropriated dialogues from political interviews with figures such as Glenn Beck, Hillary Clinton, Sarah Palin, Barack Obama and John Boehner as well as fragments of speeches by other US political leaders from the 1970s onwards. As well as appropriating such dialogues and speeches, the script interweaves citations from cultural studies texts such as Sara Ahmed's *The Cultural Politics of Emotions* as well as classic texts on rhetoric and speech-making including Delsarte's nineteenth-century analysis of everyday patterns of speech and gesture for podium and stage.[3] Hyperbolically performing the resulting speech acts as exchanges between actor couples in the audience, the work underscored how politicians' rhetorical ploys tap into the shared habitus of therapeutic discourse, especially in how the latter plays out in romantic relationships, i.e. as apologies for past offences, promises to do better and requests for understanding and forgiveness.

In mimicking these rhetorical ploys, Laser attempts to trace the symptomatology of the public sphere of politics. Rather than looking to reveal a truth, she says that: 'I'm looking at symptoms and trying to trace our way

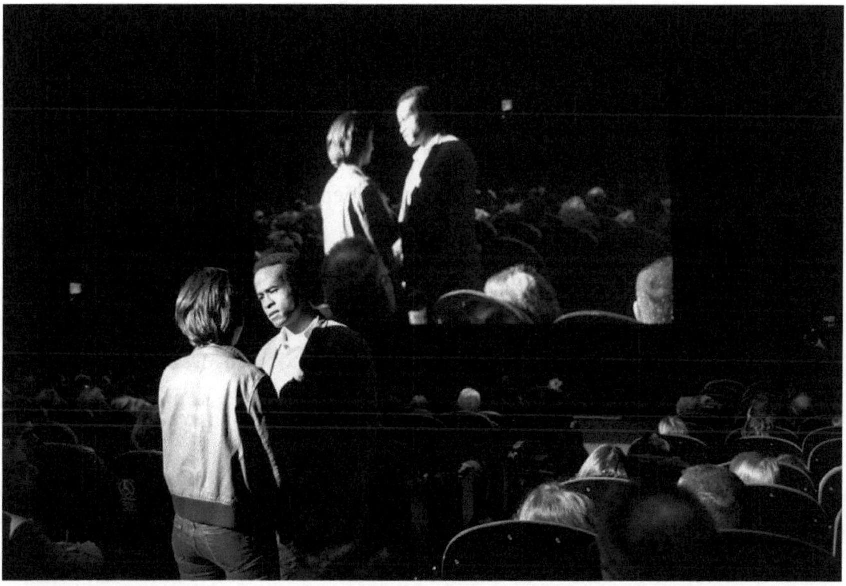

Figure 6.1 Liz Magic Laser, *I Feel Your Pain* (2011), Production Still by Yola Monakhov, Courtesy of the artist.

back to where this is coming from. That search for the authentic display is both what's driving me and what I am critiquing and reacting against' (2012).[4] In this sense then, *I Feel Your Pain* could be said to enact a kind of homeopathic mimicry of how politics is performed as emotional and therapeutic spectacle. My question is what a homeopathic aesthetic dose of the same might do to that which it sets out to critique? Is its 'cure' purely to evince a criticality premised on Shaviro's 'aesthetic inefficacy' or, conversely, the 'paranoid suspicion' that Eve Kosofsky Sedgwick claims is 'central to critical practice in the humanities'? (in Best, 2016: 3). For example, discussing the exchange between two actors that Laser modelled on a first date scenario, appropriating the flirtatious dialogue between Sarah Palin and media host Glenn Beck on a Fox News television interview in 2010, Jordan Troeller says:

> the disjunction between the generic scene before us [...] and the original context of the dialogues generates a range of emotions on the part of the audience, including amusement and discomfort, but the discomfort is instructive: in contemplating the exchange, we recognize that a crucial task of the American political system, for reporters and politicians alike, is to choreograph the emotions of the viewing public. (in Scepanski, 2014: 119)

However, as opposed to this view of a dawning critical consciousness, I would argue that the public, and undoubtedly the art world audience that attended the live performance of this work at the School of Visual Arts Theatre in New York in 2011, are well aware of how they are being manipulated by politicians.[5] But, although there is disbelief in politicians' rhetoric, there is also a sense in which, at an unconscious level, it taps into deeply held belief systems of right and wrong as well as offering the comforting illusion that there is someone in charge. It is as if emotional investments in politicians operate according to Octave Mannoni's phrase 'I know well, but all the same ... '.[6] Although Mannoni was referring to the Freudian structure of perversion, my use of it here, while not unrelated, is more prosaic: 'I know that so-and-so is a fraud, but I'm going to believe in him/her anyway, as someone else, (or something else, recalling Winnicott's fear of future catastrophe above) would be worse.' In continually confessing their problems and apologizing for mistakes in order to come across as both caring and ordinary, politicians' therapeutic emotional style distracts the public from attending to their real failures to organize and distribute resources equitably. Instead, personal moral 'failures' are framed as mistakes in the past that can be improved upon now that they have been 'openly' admitted to and witnessed by a forgiving public. In Laser's staging of the admittance that catastrophe (mistakes, failures) has already happened, there is a kind of perverse simulation of the Winnicottian notion of moving forwards towards a better future. However, a pharmacological aesthetics does more than hold a critical mirror up to society. Encapsulating the ambivalence of the pharmakon, i.e. that the same term or substance is both poison and remedy, it also facilitates the 'capacity to assimilate the consequences of destruction and violence' (Sedgwick in Best, 2016: 3)[7] without erasing them. In *I Feel Your Pain*, the performativity of apology opens up a space that hovers between these parameters.

The pharmacological aesthetics of apology

The final series of enacted vignettes in *I Feel Your Pain* focus on fantasy apologies scripted from an interview between Anthony Weiner and Arnold Schwarzenegger. The actors, in largely male and female couples, perform these apologies with increasing hysterical passion, again parodying romantic relationships as political spectacle. Stereotypically, the women perform the betrayed in the relationship, a figure who stands for the press and the public at different points in the enactment. Listening to and watching the female actors voicing betrayal is potentially agitating but the rhetoric of apology cannot move beyond its cyclical repetition. This would seem to be a good example of Shaviro's 'aesthetic inefficacy'. As opposed to the necessity for a demonstration of action to follow an apology in the political sphere, e.g. the giving or foreclosing of some kind of restitution, in the work of art, apology is poised on the brink of action. In hyperbolically performing apology, *I Feel Your Pain* could be said to suspend it precariously between perception and apprehension, a strategy Laser deploys in other works such as *The Thought Leader*, a single-channel video in which a ten-year-old actor, Alex Ammerman, delivers a satirical TED Talk. For the latter work, Ammerman stands in the centre of a parenthesis printed on a red circular rug, a prop that is a work in its own right called *Parenthesis* (2015). His speech on the theme of enlightened self-interest is based on an adaptation of Fyodor Dostoevsky's 1864 novella *Notes from the Underground*. Filmed at Kickstarters Theatre in New York in front of an audience of friends, invited actors and students, he mimics the upbeat tenor of TED Talks, yet his words and gestures generate a confusion of tongues that ultimately debases the motivational purpose of such talks. While in *The Thought Leader*, Laser empties out the persuasive efficacy of emotional rhetoric, in *I Feel Your Pain*, she exacerbates it to such an extent that it too becomes formally empty. In the final chorus of *I Feel Your Pain*, the actors perform a hysterical relay of apologies and demands for resignation that culminate in a crescendo in which 'they' take full responsibility for 'their' actions and apologize emphatically to 'the people'. The on-screen shot is a live image of the audience, who here stand in for 'the people' constantly referred to in the speeches, their image being replicated in a series of mirror projections concavely extending to infinity into the screen. A sense of pathos emerges in the exposure of gestures that are ambivalently believed in. Undoubtedly, the work performs criticality, but might there not also be an element of the restorative in *I Feel Your Pain*?

Sara Ahmed, one of Laser's citational references, has some interesting things to say about the politics of apology as both toxic and healing. Ahmed situates apology as a particular kind of performative speech act which Austin referred to as behabitives (Ahmed, 2004: 115). Unlike performatives proper, their utterance is not synonymous with the performing of an action under conditions of ritual and law. Behabitives involve the adoption of an attitude of 'seeming'. For example, apology, as Ahmed says, can be a purely rhetorical performance without being accompanied by feeling the shame of the act for which apology is being sought. In this, the behabitive speech act of apology is both slippery and generative. For Ahmed, unlike Austin, an apology can work even if the speaker does not feel sorry, as the addressee may accept the apology. And, of course, if one does genuinely feel sorry, the other may refuse the apology. This unpredictability leads Ahmed to pose the question of whether, given the unfinished nature of apology at the moment of apologizing, apology is a form of action in itself. It leaves addressees to decide whether this apology apologizes or whether it rhetorically covers over wrong-doing (115).

The closing act of *I Feel Your Pain* mimics the rhetoric of public apologies to such an extent that the audience cannot but see through the façade, but, as

I have already said, the public is well aware of the lies spouted by politicians, decisions to believe them being based on other facets of self-interest, including self-continuity or survival in order to prevent one's world from disintegrating, as I referred to above in relation to Winnicott's 'Fear of Breakdown'. However, in a theatrical setting, something more undecidable emerges in the cumulated repetition of Laser's performative apologies. Witnessing these passionately (in)sincere declarations not only makes us hyperbolically aware of their real absence in the public sphere, but, in doing so, generates a feeling, rather than a knowledge, of 'aesthetic inefficacy' which leaves us in a quandary of how to act. This might be uncomfortable, but as in Winnicott's notion of fear of breakdown, staying with that feeling can also enable us to tolerate the anxiety of what it might mean to move forwards without attachments, something that works against the vested interests of biopolitical governance. While *I Feel Your Pain* overtly uses the same kinds of linguistic tropes that circulate in the affectsphere of political spectacle, albeit to reorient them, Laser's later work, *Primal Speech*, performs a more restorative potential in its play between the cul-de-sac of 'aesthetic inefficacy' and the unpredictable outcomes that might follow from implosion. And just to reiterate that I am using the term 'restorative' here not in the sense of reinstating a stable order, but in Sedgwick's sense of reparation in which repair, always cognizant of the inherent destruction involved in any act, involves 'changing and heterogeneous relational stances' (Sedgwick 2003: 128).

Primal Speech

Primal Speech can be viewed as a single-channel, approximately twelve-minute video, but it is importantly exhibited as part of a gallery installation that includes a number of sculptural objects, grey felt 'toys' and pillows. The latter are scattered on a grey polyurethane mattress akin to the one the actors are shown to be sitting on at the end of the film.[8] Both on-screen actors and viewers have access to the grey polyurethane punching pillows, but only the viewer is surrounded by the soft 'toys', which are key to my pharmacological interpretation of the work in what follows. The video features six actors, one of whom directs the group using techniques based on Arthur Janov's primal-scream therapy, a radical 1970s therapeutic approach that used 'abreaction', i.e. the cathartic re-experiencing of a traumatic or repressed event, as a way of discharging its negative effects on one's life. In this method, a therapist would coach patients to re-enact scenes from their past and express repressed feelings with the aim of liberating them from the repetition of unhealthy behaviours. This form of therapy is deemed highly dubious due to its relation to the counter-cultural, often drug-fuelled, spiritual ethos of 'letting it all hang out' and its potentially exploitative investment in the unsubstantiated belief that the body stores traumatic memory intact and that this can be exorcized by extreme forms of acting-out. Rather than an endorsement of this therapeutic practice, *Primal Speech* deploys it as a technique to examine the structural fantasies that underlie toxic political belief systems. To this end, Laser collaborated with Valerie Bell, a certified professional life coach trained in primal therapy techniques, to engage actors to perform the conflictual emotions generated by political events that coincided with the execution of the work, for example the US presidential election in 2016 and the UK referendum on Brexit in 2017. Casting actors who had strong political beliefs, Laser describes seeking out people 'who would allow me to conflate their personal traumas with their political frustrations' (Laser in Kiefer, 2016: 82).

> I explained to them beforehand that the project would involve primal therapy, a radical therapeutic method from the '70s that focused on abreaction: the cathartic re-experiencing of a traumatic event. In this method the therapist is much more active, more like a director. Once they get a patient to start talking about how they were abused as a child, for instance, they almost hypnotize them into reliving that memory. I was interested in its similarity to Stanislavski's concept of emotional memory, which became the basis for method acting. (Laser in Kiefer: 84–5)

Interestingly, Stanislavski's idea that an actor should regress to the past to find an experience so as to act out a required emotion in the present, a process combatted by the historical avant-garde such as Brecht due to its problematic naturalism, is now being used to train politicians and business leaders to increase their persuasiveness. As Laser describes it: 'The same performance methods used to conjure audience empathy are being applied in tandem with market research to engineer public opinion' (Laser in Steffen, 2011: 105). Interested in 'how market research and therapy both use discourse as a "treatment"' (in Kiefer: 82), Laser's work hovers on the boundary of being purely critical and being more pharmacologically driven in advocating a certain salutary inflection of therapeutic aesthetics. In what follows, I want to explore the latter impetus in relation to the space of object-testing derived from Winnicott's transitional phenomenon, but this time, rather than Stiegler's deconstructive reading of the pharmakon as poison and cure in the transitional space of audio-visual environments, I turn to psychoanalyst and theorist Juliet Mitchell's notion of shifting from 'identicality' to 'separation' which I categorize as the development of the capacity to tolerate anxiety.

Primal Speech opens with a direct-to-camera close-up of the therapist Ghisla Chípe, whose soothing adjuration to relax, to 'check in with your feelings', think about the latest news and how it makes you feel, immediately incorporates the viewer into the scenario.[9] When the therapist asks her clients to locate their feelings in their body, in their jaw, chest and belly, I myself began to perform the kinds of inner adjustments characteristic of meditation or yoga classes. In this, I was being a good subject of cognitive capitalism, renewing my energy to enhance my productivity; subjecting to my neuromobilization, as Berardi might put it. Although, of course, I did not experience the abreactive catharsis feigned by the other five actors, the clients, I did feel momentarily more relaxed as a result of going through this simulated group therapy. However, as opposed to this one-dimensional approach to the work, the pharmacological nature of its aesthetics is more ambivalent, both in its use of therapeutic discourse to critique political spectacle and to suggest a way of bypassing its interpellation of the public.

Following the opening instructions, the video cuts to a close-up of a mixed-race actor lying on a padded cushion, who confesses to being marginalized and bullied in his life. His personal reflections quickly segue into a rant about how Donald J. Trump is a bully led by fear and hate to incite violence. The scene shifts to another isolated figure, an older white man, the montage suggesting he might be lying opposite the first actor, though there is no dialogue between them. The older man asserts his identification with Trump as a stand-up guy who has been misunderstood as a populist. The actors' diametrically opposed political opinions conflate politicians with paternal/parental figures who they either love or hate, the polarities cutting across racial and sexual – though not class – lines. A seemingly, well-heeled, mixed-race woman voices her anger with people blindly supporting Trump, followed by a young English white woman who voices her sadness at being 'shut out of Europe' due to the recent Brexit poll in the UK, while a black woman of similar age sees Brexit as a chance for people to take back power. The viewer oscillates between these diametric opposites, agreeing or disagreeing, identifying or dis-identifying, the conflict exacerbated by the emotional outbursts into more personal terrain that equate political betrayal to betrayal by intimate others. Elaborating on these binaries in an interview discussion, Laser and Keefer (2016) refer to conservative cognitive linguist and philosopher George P. Lakoff's thesis that the basis for our concept of proper government is a deeply internalized idea about the nuclear family in which the father role is premised on either a strict punitive or a nurturing parent model, identification with either setting the ground for later political affiliation. This splitting is echoed by political splits in society between Right and Left, Laser being particularly interested in how the Right use market research to tap into emotional concerns such as the fear that freedom and liberty are being taken away from them and doled out to disenfranchised groups. The actors' dichotomous belief systems mirror these societal and political binaries.

On the one hand, the work performs the attempt to exorcize the disabling emotions which are generated by political events over which we have no control and which reduce us to political spectators whose actions are often ignored, e.g. the massive anti-war protests in London in 2003 against joining forces with the United States in the Iraq War which were ignored by the then UK Labour government. In real life, people resolve conflictual emotion by choosing one side over another and making hard and fast rules about what is right and wrong, such categorizations often resulting in violence, racism and hate speech. *Primal Speech* proposes another form of resolution, a therapeutic suspension of action, yet another kind of parenthesis as in her previous work. But perhaps something else also begins to emerge in this space.

The video continuously cuts between close-ups of Chípe instructing her clients 'to vent their anger at figures in the media that enrage them' and close-ups of them expressing their rage, but edited so that they appear to be in individual therapy sessions. Therefore, it is a surprise when the middle-distance shot at the end of *Primal Speech* reveals the actors together in the

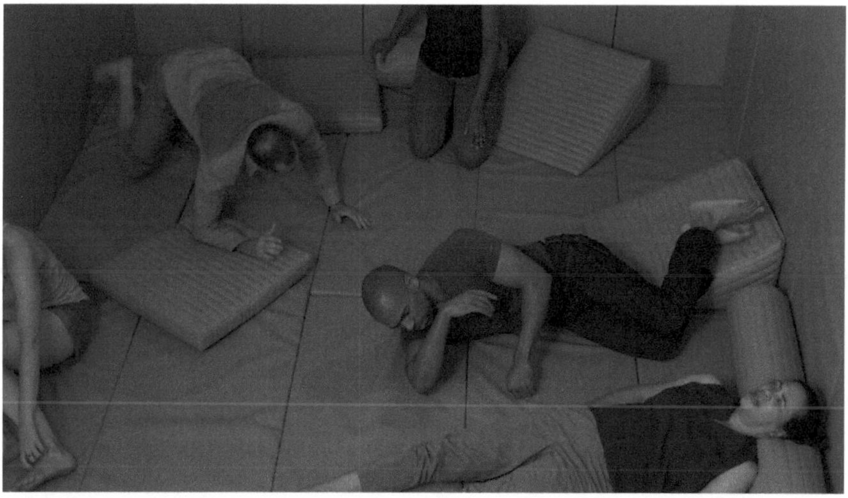

Figure 6.2 Liz Magic Laser, *Primal Speech* (2016), video still, Courtesy of the artist.

same grey padded room, all coiling in on themselves in various post-rage positions. There is no solidarity here, Laser's video suggesting that the acting out of emotional fear and rage stemming from betrayal and abuse leads to an exhausted and individualized acquiescence. Is this a retreat from the political and a reversion to a self-enclosed subjectivity or might this group 'exhaustion' be the ground of a new solidarity as some political philosophers, such Berardi, posit?

As I mentioned in the previous chapter, Berardi calls for the withdrawal of cognitive productivity from the cognitive capitalist sphere of 'neuromobilization and compulsory creativity' (2011: 36). Exhaustion and depression are two of the modes of withdrawal that Berardi claims as having some political purchase in resisting the co-option of body and soul in neoliberal cognitive capitalism. Not only this, but he also advocates the therapeutic as a modality of going beyond a merely negative withdrawal saying that:

> Politics and therapy will be one and the same activity in the coming years. People will feel hopeless and depressed and panicky because they are unable to deal with the post-growth economy, and because they will miss their dissolving modern identity. Our cultural task will be attending to those people and taking care of their insanity, showing them the way to a happy adaptation. (2011: 153)

Jason Smith interprets Berardi's notion of adaptation as the generation of a common sensibility, a communalist approach to 'the post-political era [that] opens not onto an administration of things [...] but to what is here daringly called *therapy* – that is, with the articulation of "happy singularizations" that defect from the metropolitan factory of unhappiness' (Smith in Berardi, 2009: 17). Although this sounds rather vague, I nonetheless find it a productive metaphor of how to rethink the implosive withdrawal in *Primal Speech* as itself a moment in such a process of re-singularization which Smith refers to as 'primarily aesthetic in nature' (19).

At one level, the video seems to propose an adaptation to the disappointments in leaders and intimate others, compensated for by having the social capital to be able to articulate this disappointment and anger in the terms and context of therapeutic discourse. The problem with such a use of therapeutic discourse is that it risks adapting to what Furedi calls the 'depoliticised language of managerialism' (2004: 54). Managerialism encourages its subjects to be productive, flexible and creative in relation to adapting to the constant procedural change that is a feature of the contemporary workplace. Although self-supporting networks can and do form around negative emotions such as depression and low self-esteem, therapeutic discourse encourages subjects to manage their feelings so as to achieve positive goal-oriented outcomes in relation to such changes. In Furedi's sociological critique: 'Therapeutics is oriented to the experience of the atomised individual and tries to give meaning to the experience of isolated alienation' (2004: 89). Although he is writing over a decade ago, his reference to the script of the self as enforcing a lack of solidarity that extends across all spectrums of society (91) would seem to be apropos in relation to Laser's video. For Furedi, the therapeutic outlook 'threatens to displace politics' (50), public emoting being encouraged the more that public resources are privatized. His thesis, which I agree with, is that 'we' are governed using counselling technologies that have seeped into the general atmosphere of institutional establishments whether or not we are on the receiving end of actual therapy (61). Governmental exhortations to well-being treat its population (I am referring specifically to the UK as that is the context I am familiar with),[10] as subjects who are vulnerable and at risk, yet its policies and corporate affiliations result in generating even more anxiety for its citizens. At the same time as being assured that our leaders can and want to protect us, we are also told that it is our responsibility to achieve productive, successful and healthy lives. The main thrust of therapeutic emotional style is empathy, not judgement (Furedi, 2004: 97), as the self is considered too vulnerable to be judged but yet, on the other hand, that very self is exhorted to achieve an autonomy in which responsibility for oneself is key to success, or even survival. *Primal Speech* performs the duplicity of managing personal survival in a toxic environment via the catharsis of conflictual emotion, a process that entails the suppression of anger, a well-known motivator of political change. While therapeutic, confessional, discourse may be a useful framework in which to narrate one's personal feelings of oppression and anger vis-à-vis governing power structures, these outpourings are not only easily accommodated within those very structures, but required by them as evidence that our personal feelings are being taken into account. This paradox is well articulated by Illouz in *Cold Intimacies* in which she asserts that, while emoting in institutional life is of value to the self, this emotional openness is also a means of further subjection. So, on one level, *Primal Speech* performs how therapeutic narratives enable an adaptation to things as they are perceived to be, the use of performative play in the work drawing attention to how the acting-out of individual choices and problems ultimately results in a cycle of implosion and recuperation. The outcome of the final scene in *Primal Speech* is each to their own remedy which, as Jonathan Beller (2006) paraphrasing Marx claims, enables you to function in the morning and produce more value for the capitalist machine.

However, and this is the work's pharmacological aesthetics, the performative implosion also suggests (and the workshops seem to substantiate this), the necessity of admitting that you cannot cope with political events over which you have no control.[11] This might be a step towards another kind of withdrawal in which those who have nothing in common might nonetheless find a kind of solidarity. While theorists such as Slavoj Žižek make sweeping statements that capitalism works because we all subscribe to it without believing in it (in Fisher 2009: 13), it is also crucial to find ways of surviving within a system that works against the majority of people. This does not mean necessarily ascribing to dominant values, but of finding ways to negotiate existence on terms other than the cynical or ironic. That said, Berardi's call for a 'happy adaptation' that, as Smith articulates it, involves 'the composition of a *refrain* that constitutes a territory subtracted from the social factory and its temporalities and rhythms' (in Berardi 2009: 19) is not available to many. Most people do not have the option of such a retreat from corporate or institutional life, but this does not mean they do not find their own ways of flourishing beyond a mere capitulation to consumerist political ideology.[12]

As I watched the video in the installation, I absentmindedly pulled the felt 'toys' closer, their tactility and scale incongruously appealing. Given the crudeness of their shapes, at first, I did not connect them to the actual symbols they are based on, but to more generic animal and plant hybrid figures. In fact, the 'toys' are crudely sewn in the shape of the symbols of political parties: an oak tree for Conservative; a donkey for Democrat; a rose for socialist; flames for the National Front and an elephant for Republican. However, I did not feel by handling these objects that I was subscribing to a political party. Nor did I feel I had been duped when I found out their derivation. By contrast, the sculptural aspect of the work extended the video's therapeutic scene into a transitional space in which the meaning of objects could be puzzled over rather than predetermined by political symbolism and its congruent affiliation. For example, the shape of the 'elephant' was suggestive of a kind of palm tree or organic growth rather than an elephant per se. The set-up of the installation alludes to Winnicott's intermediate area of experience but, in Winnicott's psychoanalytic version, objects take on an idiosyncratic symbolic value between the real and the imaginary, not a literal value as in Laser's intentions. However, to me, the crudity of the shapes displaced their overt semiology. The supposed oak tree could be a fish; the flames, leaves; the fist and rose, a weird animal. Importantly, the actors in the video, who are proxies for possible viewers, do not have access to these objects. In this transitional space of symbolic over-determination, the experience of the installation of *Primal Speech* is more expansive than the video alone. The conjunction of handling the 'toys' while witnessing the oscillatory dynamic between oppositional political viewpoints might enable a gallery audience to test out different imaginative possibilities. If we think of Lakoff's aforementioned, somewhat simplistic, but nonetheless productive, notion that political discourse operates by using simple metaphors that tap into identifications based on parental repressive or permissive modalities, then a technique for alleviating the familiar pathways of this feedback circuit is potentially productive. While my methodology is not psychoanalytic, Winnicott's transitional space is relevant here, not only because it is the nexus through which Stiegler weaves his pharmacological argument about the poisonous, yet curative, aspects of technology, but also because it is a potential space in which nourishing pleasures can be accessed in simultaneity with toxic ones, the boundaries between them being unstable.

To further this discussion of the ambivalence of transitional space, I now want to turn to a reading of Winnicott's work by feminist psychoanalyst Juliet Mitchell that appeared in the art history journal *October* in 2005. Mitchell focuses on Winnicott's 'The Use of an Object and Relating through Identifications'[13] which situates his concept of the transitional object in relation to the problematic of identification, which for me is a pharmacological question in that its hold on the subject leads to toxic relations that while pleasurable are hard to let go of. Laser's *Primal Speech* pivots around the issue of identification and whether its primary grip might be released a little in order to enable a creative flourishing, rather than a dogged, repetition of the same. Transitional phenomena are crucial for the withdrawal of a form of identification that Mitchell calls 'identicality' (Mitchell, 2005: 34). 'Identicality' is what ties mother and child or parent and child to an unconscious identification based on a similarity between them to the exclusion of difference. They are tied, Mitchell says, to the same feelings, an attachment that is comforting but also frustrating as it does not allow the 'child' its separate existence. Enter the transitional object. The transitional object contains the infant's frustrations with these feelings without completely destroying them. (To utterly destroy them would be to disable sociality.) In allowing itself to be destroyed and thereby 'used' by the infant, the transitional object effects a psychic destruction of this primal attachment *without cutting off all ties with it*. It is in this sense that the transitional object is pharmacological. It retains the toxicity of destruction and engulfment triggered by 'identicality' in conjunction with the pleasure of finding likeness in the world, at the same time as it effects a separation from them. The potentiality of transitional space enables the externalization of attachments so that they become objects to be 'used', i.e. destroyed in fantasy, and moved away from without feelings of abandonment. Although there are gendered aspects to this – Mitchell refers to the mother as the one from whom separation is necessary, while Laser and Keefer refer to paternal figures – my argument is the more general one of how the transitional object facilitates the infant to shift from 'identicality' into 'separation', i.e. a space in which new thoughts might come into being. This is not a comfortable space, thinking in psychoanalysis being fraught with the anxiety of separation, which, however, one must learn to tolerate to prevent regression to an unthinking 'identicality'.

The obverse of 'separation' is acted out in Laser's script. When political 'identicality' is threatened, the actors resort to projecting parental imagos that they accuse of abandonment. For example, in the monologue of the man who reproaches his idol, Trump, for not protecting him from the manipulative vagaries of his Russian girlfriend, the boundaries between Trump and a parental father figure become blurred. The man's breakdown – as evidenced by profuse sweating and an exhibition of vulnerability – ends with an entropic withdrawal into the self. This is akin to the 'aesthetic inefficacy' of Shaviro's aesthetics of acceleration. However, as Berardi, in his critique of acceleration, says: 'acceleration is provoking an impoverishment of the experience, as the intensive modalities of pleasure and knowledge are stressed up to the point of exhaustion' (2015: 37). For Berardi, exhaustion can also be used positively as a withdrawal of energy from the cognitive capitalist ethos of competition and progress, and, therefore potentially, a mode of 'separation'. In fact, Berardi sees emotional states such as depression as a positive force that teaches one to look for meaning in life outside of the prevailing social and political environment. The psychoanalytic counterpart to this would be that 'separation' too involves a necessary sadness that arises from the knowledge that while 'identicality' is pleasurable, it is also harmful. While at the end of Laser's video, there is no escape from individualistic isolation, the 'aesthetic inefficacy' that ensues as a result of performed abreaction could be argued to be poised on the brink of 'separation', i.e. the moving away from inhibiting and subjugating ideas towards an undecidable outcome.

My speculation that *Primal Speech* proposes a move away from the 'identicality' of political identification and into something like 'separation', i.e. a space in which new thoughts might come into being, is predicated on the ambiguity of the 'toys'. In conjunction with the life coach's soothing tones, they become objects to be 'used', aesthetically rather than instrumentally, in the parenthesis left open by the actors' withdrawal into themselves. No artwork can solve social problems, but the enactment of imaginative propositions can be real in art. This might be the beginnings of a therapeutic aesthetics as distinct from 'prevailing techniques of therapy [that] are aimed to adapt the suffering organism to the social and technical environment' (Berardi in de Boever and Neidich, 2013: 19). In becoming an object to be used, *Primal Speech* might move its viewer from the comforting subjection of 'identicality' towards a feeling of being able to tolerate the anxiety of 'separation' without the need for an apology.

7

Leigh Ledare's pharmacological aesthetics of group analysis

In this chapter I shall continue to explore the moving image artwork as a transitional space that potentially enables participants, both on- and off-screen, to test out and circumnavigate identity as a mode of subjectivation, i.e. the means by which people enact their agency (Lazzarato, 2014a). While subjectivation involves subjugation to the environment in which one is embedded, individuals are not reducible to this subjection. As I outlined in the previous chapter in relation to Winnicott's spheres of 'identicality' and 'separation', intersubjective relations are determined by the transitional environment yet are also distinct from it due to the singularity of the transitional object as a phenomenologically complex entity, it being both real and virtual and neither fully within nor without. As Stiegler, in his adoption of Winnicott, interprets it: 'beyond that part of the object that exists in external space, beyond or beneath this piece of cloth, there holds something that is precisely neither in external space, nor simply internal to either the mother or the child' (Stiegler, 2013a: 2). This is the pharmacological dimension of being which is opened up by the object that appears on the child's mental horizon. The child's internalization of this object, which for Stiegler is the technical object, can engage 'not only curative projection processes but poisonous ones' (2013a: 3), the problem, as he identifies it, being that this process of internalization is increasingly channelled by the audio-visual environment towards toxic consumption. Also, being captured in the specular economy of the audio-visual involves the subjection of persons to identitarian categories that may harm – think of how certain (raced and gendered) bodies are coded as being dangerous and/or threatening. However, my wager in this book is that technologies of capture can also be used by 'actants' to reconfigure their subjectivity in autonomous (curative) ways.[1]

My main case study in this chapter will be Leigh Ledare's staged documentary films, *The Large Group (Zurich)* (2016) and *The Task* (2017), in which scenarios based on the Tavistock Institute's method of group analysis are enacted.[2] This method of group analysis is grounded in the theories of psychoanalyst Wilfred Bion. I shall say more about them later in this chapter, but for now I want to note that, rather than applying these theories to moving image artworks, my focus is on how an artist might appropriate them for more pharmacological purposes. As a preamble to discussing Ledare's work, I want to briefly allude to two different kinds of practices in which technologies of capture are used for more overtly therapeutic ends. While their more positive therapeutic outcomes loosen the imbrication of poison and cure that is central to my main argument, they nonetheless suggest an interrelation between the projected image of capture and those captured that sets a useful context for Ledare's pharmacological aesthetics.

Two different kinds of practices: A preamble

My first example is the photo therapy work developed by Jo Spence together with Rosy Martin in their collaboration *Phototherapy* (1984–1986).[3] While this is not moving image work, it shares its photographic basis. Photo therapy, as developed by Spence and Martin in 1983, grew out of the practice of co-counselling that both artists were involved in at the time.[4] The process of photo therapy involved the artists enacting various stereotypes of women from their cultural image repertoires as well as restaging childhood photographs. In the course of their sessions, the roles of being behind the camera and in front of the camera would be exchanged between them. Their performances-to-camera, captured in what were originally printed as snapshots, were bookended by pre-shoot discussions lasting an hour or so in which one would listen to and encourage the other, and post-shoot discussions between themselves as well as with their peer group. The images were exhibited alongside accompanying text explaining their process of 'reframing', a co-counselling technique that was the impetus for the practice:

> We take a specific piece of behaviour, history, or in this case an image, examine what it represents to us and how we would like to change it – that

> is, change our impression of what we think about it. Put crudely, reframing is a kind of internal permission-giving: permission to change, to re-view, to let go, to move on. It is not a way of discussing the 'real' in order to see if it is 'biased' but of finding new ways of perceiving the past so that we can change our activities now. Through the medium of visual reframing we can begin to see that images we hold of ourselves are often the embodiment of particular traumas, fears, losses, hopes and desires. (Martin and Spence, 1985: 67)

Through dialogue and performative play, the process of 'reframing' provides new inhabitations of parental imagos and other identitarian categories rather than fixed images of representation. As Martin says: 'this kind of working together [was] not like looking in the mirror' (in Martin and Spence, 1985: 68). Rather than a re-soldering of self and image, the process of working was to interpret and discuss the projection of what it felt like to performatively embody pre-existing images, whether these be personal photographs or social stereotypes of women as well as female mythic archetypes. Idealized images in personal childhood photographs were also reclaimed and recreated, Martin's stated goal being 'to reach a balanced state that recognises and integrates strength and vulnerability, independence and dependence, and to accept that both aspects co-exist' (in Martin and Spence, 1985: 73). In the same article, Spence describes how, in a session of working on a school photograph that was a site of trauma for her, the collaborative *movement through* visual memories of self and parents ended up with a more joyful transformation – my emphasis. In this use of photography as a transitional space of circumnavigating identity, the artists sometimes performatively exacerbated trauma in order to move into this more joyful space (1985: 75). The traumas do not change, but how they think about them does. While this shares some of the goals of contemporary forms of CBT, the latter is more focused on personal responsibility and societal adaptation rather than the performative play with trauma that Martin and Spence enacted in their collaborative photographic practice. My interest in recounting this example for what follows is in how the camera serves as an interface that both draws out the artists' performances and projects them as objects that can be used to generate new circuits of exchange between the artists, in the first place, and, later, their peer review group and perhaps further audiences. The machinic gaze of the camera acts like a transitional space in which boundaries between the self and the social can be tested and renegotiated. As Martin puts it: 'the objectifying eye of the camera offers a blank screen and the necessary distance to see from a different point-of-view' (in Loewenthal, 2013: 77).[5]

My second example relates to the use of video by Carry Gorney, currently a systemic psychotherapist and writer, who worked in community arts video projects in London in the 1960s and 1970s, as well as in Milton Keynes, a town north-west of London. Gorney used a dialogic process to make the community arts film *Women Talking* (1978). Initial filming involved Gorney encouraging the women who lived on new estates in Milton Keynes to talk about their lives as mothers and wives. The results were shown to the group and Gorney would let them run with it, future filming sessions being informed by the women's projections of how they perceived and reflected on the initial footage. As she describes it:

> Once they watched themselves on video, their conversation would take the discussion up to another level. They would say things like: 'I wouldn't have been single then, but maybe I'd have chosen to do it at a different time'. They would become less clichéd about it, more reflective, thinking more and not just saying something sensational for the camera. (in Waller, 2011)

Gorney went on to work for the NHS, pioneering the use of video in therapeutic settings to enable young parents' confidence through the 'Seeing Is Believing' programme.[6] This involved Gorney filming interaction between mother and infant, then editing the positive moments which would be projected and discussed with the mothers in further therapeutic sessions. What interests me about this programme and *Women Talking*, and what I want to feed into my discussion of Ledare's work, is how the camera's neutral gaze and technological capacity capture aspects of behaviour that are invisible to the naked eye, operating as they do beneath human consciousness. When projected, the potentially transformative gestures captured at this unconscious level can be recognized and thereby capitalized on to generate future behaviours. In *Women Talking*, the women were able to use their perceptions of themselves in the feedback screenings to project their desires and ideas forwards into future filming sessions. And in the parenting therapeutic sessions, the video image enabled mothers who thought they were unable to parent, and were considered at risk, to perceive a different story. In conjunction with Gorney's encouragement, the mothers come to observe that they have skills they are unaware of, this perception giving them confidence to build future behaviour based on the positive expressions of care captured by the camera. This capacity of documentary-style moving image to capture the micro-movements of unconscious gestures that are unavailable to conscious reflection is reminiscent of Walter Benjamin's notion of film as an optical unconscious.[7] Interestingly, in an article co-written by four clinicians at Sheffield CAMHS, including Gorney, they remark that 'the microanalysis of video frames holds time still', thereby allowing that which goes unnoticed to be perceived (in Pearlman et al., 2013: 23). The gestural attunement that happens between parents and infant would be lost to consciousness unless mediated by the camera, its projection having a life-enhancing effect on future behaviour. However, my interest is less with the therapeutic goal of clinical work than with how the technological apparatus of the camera provides an interface that acts as a 'feed-forward structure' projecting behavioural enactments that might transform life.

I am appropriating the notion of 'feed-forward structure' from Mark B.N. Hansen (2015: 77). In his take up of Stiegler's technics to explore the potential of the digital to enhance subjectivity, Hansen proffers the pharmacological view that, on the one hand, this enhancement 'has been left to capitalist culture to exploit [and] create closed loop circuits between the past behaviour of consumers and their probable future activity' (2015: 70). However, on the other hand, the capacity of digital technology to tap into what he calls the 'microtemporal technics that operate beneath human consciousness' (2015: 79) can also be used to get out of such closed loop circuits, creating instead 'a feed-forward structure' (77). For Hansen, digital technology works with what he calls, following Maurice Merleau-Ponty, the interoceptive phenomenal body (24). In Merleau-Ponty's phenomenology, the interoceptive body always has a capacity for sensory perception and apprehension that exceeds the specular. While Hansen focuses specifically on the machinic environments of the digital, for me, the concept of a 'feed-forward structure' can equally serve as a metaphor of how older technologies of capture such as film and video might be said to constitute environments that bypass subjection to the capitalist attention economy. My argument is that, in facilitating feedback between the various 'actors' and/or 'actants' enmeshed in an audio-visual environment, Ledare's moving image artworks make available performances that are invisible to the naked eye, a process that is key to informing subjectivation beyond mere subjection to the apparatus.

Leigh Ledare's pharmacological aesthetics

It could be said that the transformative nature of Ledare's work is more questionable than the aforementioned examples and that his therapeutic theatres exacerbate the tensile condition of being a body in a specular social field of relations, albeit intentionally. Situated in relation to the ubiquity of surveillance and social media, as well as his own proclivities in using the inherent voyeurism of the camera to question the contractual nature of interpersonal relationships, his work addresses the more poisonous side of pharmacological therapeutics in relation to moving image technology. Nonetheless, in prefacing his documentary-style moving image artworks with the more overtly therapeutic examples above, I claim that his toxic exacerbation of interpersonal relations might also be seen as inadvertently life-enhancing. Ledare's *The Large Group (Zurich)* and *The Task* both assemble voluntary non-professional actor participants to partake in sessions based on the Tavistock Method of group analysis but under Ledare's observation in conjunction with the mediation of the camera apparatus. A unique social experiment, Ledare's work could be said to have some commonality with so-called relational art practices as defined by Nicolas Bourriaud rather than with social art practices in which artists insert themselves into other people's lives and/or social systems to work on transformative community projects. Bourriaud defines relational aesthetics in art as 'an activity consisting in producing relationships with the world with the help of songs, forms, actions and objects' (2002: 17). However, as opposed to Bourriaud's utopian belief that the mere fact of coming together in relational art is meaningful in itself rather than simply augmenting opportunities for collective consumption by aestheticizing, as Hal Foster puts it, 'the nicer procedures of our service economy' (in Bishop, 2006: 195), Ledare's work is much more ambivalent. His moving image artworks mirror the social milieu in ways that leave open how viewers, including the on-screen participants, might reflect on the relation between projection and behavioural enaction in group dynamics. As well as this, any 'knowledge' gleaned from this reflection cannot be reified as a method to be applied to contexts outside of its contractual on-screen enactment. While participants' post-participation experience may reverberate further in their lives, what happens in the group is intrinsic to the art situation.

The Large Group (Zurich) documents one of the group encounter sessions which was part of Ledare's larger collaboration with group therapist and specialist in childhood and adolescent psychiatry, and psychotherapy, Dr Christoph Müller. It was exhibited at Manifesta 11 in Zurich in 2016. Ledare's exhibition entitled *The Here and the Now [Zurich 1:1]* was shown across two venues, *The Large Group* at Helmhaus, while at Zürcher Hochschule der Künste, Ledare presented vitrines of the participants' own written anticipations and assessments of the process as well as his diary-like notes. The overall collaboration, of which this film was an outcome, was a three-day immersive psychology experiment involving twenty-one Zurich residents of different ages and from different walks of life in which they participated in workshops based on the London Tavistock Institute's group dynamic therapy model. However, my analysis is dependent on viewing the film as a single-screen work online.[8] As I have said, Tavistock Method has its roots in the theoretical ideas of British psychoanalyst Bion, which have been expanded on by the Tavistock Institute of Human Relations and the Tavistock Clinic in London in applications in the field of social research and group and organizational psychodynamics.[9] Prior to the film, the participants had engaged in smaller groups, each of which was led by a Tavistock-trained psychotherapist, Müller himself leading one of the groups as well as advising on the project in general. In *The Large Group*, all twenty-one participants, including three of the psychotherapists, referred to as 'consultants', come together for the first time.

The participants take up seats pre-arranged in loose concentric circles, the three 'consultants', two women and one man, only being identifiable by red badges. Not having an agenda or script, the sense of embarrassment and unease is palpable as they all look around the room wondering what to say. To break the ice, they begin by discussing what they share in common, that is, the fact that Ledare is absent, an observation which is initially misheard by some group members as being 'wine is missing', a slip of the tongue that the consultants hone in on as intimating a group desire for less 'tightness'. ('Tightness' is occasionally returned to at various points in the film, the group identifying it as a Swiss character trait.) Although the film edit does not show his entry, shortly afterwards Ledare is glimpsed on-screen sitting in the outer circle of the group watching intently as if in a mirror relation to the viewer on the other side of the screen.

Infamous for his portraits of his stripper mother posing provocatively for the camera, this work, and the subsequent *The Task*, an elaborate staging of a Tavistock group relations conference involving thirty-four participants, are less about Ledare jumping on a therapeutic bandwagon and more about a continuation of his interest in 'issues of contract, exchange, and power dynamics' (Indrisek, 2011: 49). One of his notes in the vitrines at Manifesta read, 'the group serves as a mother', which not only references his previous work but also indicates Bion's theories on which Tavistock group dynamic therapy is based. For Bion, the mother contains the infant's feelings of frustration by not reacting to them, but by returning them to the infant in a manageable, contained, state, which enables the infant to process them. While I do not want to persist with the mother motif in what follows, as my focus is on the group dynamic in Ledare's films, it is clear that the consultants act somewhat as such a figure. Bion published *Experiences in Groups* (1961) early in his career and, although his analysis of group dynamics was preliminary, it has had much impact in this psychoanalytic community whose practice is undergirded by the object relations tradition stemming from Melanie Klein.

Bion proffered that there were two kinds of group dynamics, both of which can be operative within a group, although usually one type predominates at one given time. He identified these dynamics as 'group-work mentality' and 'basic-assumption mentality and functioning'. While both are ways that groups manage shared anxieties, the former leads to a capacity for realistic hard work dependent on co-operation, whereas the latter is caught in unconscious group collusion that leads to stagnation (French and Simpson, 2010: 1859). Examples of such collusions might be dependence (on a leader, or on the group per se); pairings (between small groups within a group); and fight or flight reactions. Importantly, these formulations can sometimes lead to a 'group-work mentality', e.g. positive pairing can inspire a group to unite (French and Simpson, 2010: 1869), but, for the most part, purposive action does not occur in a group caught up in 'basic-assumption mentality and functioning'. While the latter kind of groups can appear very active, this activity serves to mask the fact that they are not united at the level of the unconscious and are actually operating 'off-purpose' (French and Simpson, 2010: 1863). Bion wrote less about 'group-work mentality'. However, citing Bion, French and Simpson proffer that this group dynamic provides a 'creative space, in which " 'thoughts' in search of a thinker" can be found and formed' (French and Simpson, 2010: 1867). This allusion to an expansive creative space in 'group-work mentality' could be said to be akin to the transitional environment that Winnicott and Stiegler see the mother as facilitating, but here mapped onto the group.

Searching for a project that might unite them, various members of the group raise interpersonal issues based on projections and prejudices

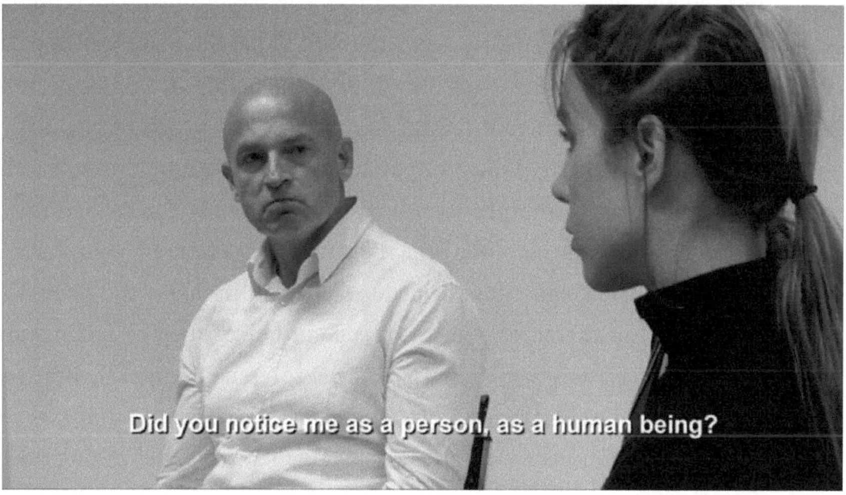

Figure 7.1 Leigh Ledare *The Large Group (Zurich)*, 2016. Courtesy of the artist.

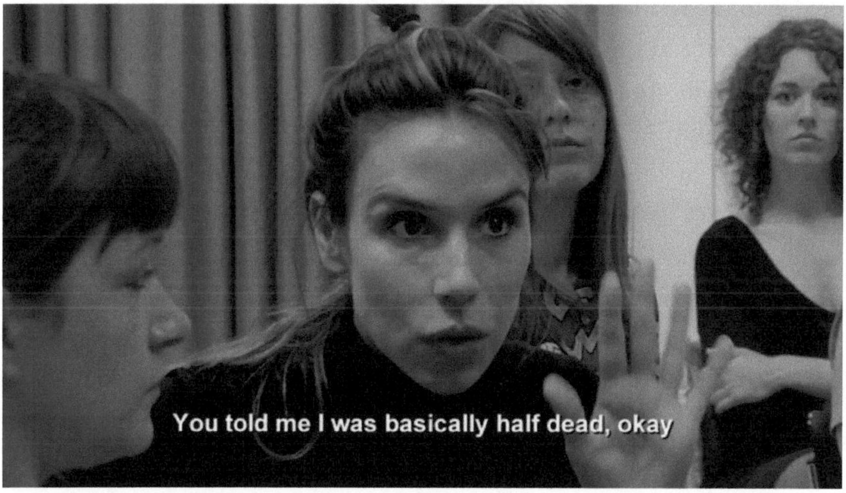

Figure 7.2 Leigh Ledare *The Large Group (Zurich)*, 2016. Courtesy of the artist.

encountered at previous meetings either in the small group sessions or in the canteen facilities provided for the three-day event. The sparring between a man from the Balkans and the young Swiss woman sitting near him becomes the focus of the group, the pair's antagonism towards each other in turn creating other pairings within the group. Given that this group encounter is being witnessed by and performed to the camera, it is interesting that what prompts their sparring is the man's accusation that the woman does not look at him directly, thereby withholding the interpersonal recognition he desires. Two other women who, prior to the film, had had antagonistic encounters with said young Swiss woman now side with her against the man. In this part of the film, the viewer could be said to observe the acting out of aspects of Bion's 'basic-assumption mentality and functioning' in which antagonistic pairings block the potential of the group to do productive group-work, which in this case might be to modify the superegoic demands for recognition. Added to this, from the outset of the film, the young Swiss woman 'voluntarily' takes on the role of scapegoat for the group, self-identifying as the one who is truly experiencing the emotional resonance of being open to feelings of vulnerability, a declaration that is itself a passive aggressive form of accusation towards the group. She gets more and more upset, but unlike as in *The Task* in which an American-Chinese woman takes up a similar role, her crying does not lead to the group using her as a mascot of victimization that distracts from other micro-aggressions that may be occurring in its environs. This may be due to the relative lack of diversity in *The Large Group* by contrast to the ethnic, racial and gender tensions in *The Task* which seem to precipitate the urgency of allocating a scapegoat to prevent the group from imploding. I will say more about *The Task* later.

However, in *The Large Group*, a shift occurs in the distribution of anxiety and imaginary projection between group members such that something like a 'group-work mentality' emerges. However, rather than Bion, I want to consider Ledare's experiments with group behaviour in the light of Félix Guattari's theories of group subjectivity. The latter somewhat echo Bion's but have the added advantage of adapting Winnicott's concept of the transitional object as a mediating object in group contexts rather than simply in a maternal-environment. Guattari refers to the transitional object as the institutional object. Specifically referring to Guattari's innovative approach to group therapy,

Gary Genosko states that the institutional object 'represents all the phenomena associated with contextualizing the psychotherapeutic cure and foregrounding the environment' (in Guattari 2000: 114). For Guattari, the group context facilitates the exteriorization of internal psychic processes so that they can be redistributed or, as Genosko puts it, 'deindividuated and depersonalized' (Genosko in Guattari, 2000: 114). In other words, they are shared across the group. For Guattari, such 'a group-subject' has the potential to evade capture by dominant power, an idea that also featured in Melanie Gilligan's exploration of collective subjectivity in Chapter 5. Guattari states that groups have the potential to *institute* themselves rather than accept predetermined structures, a modification that implies 'a takeover – even if partial – of local politics by a group-subject' (Guattari, 2009: 146). It is important to note that Guattari's reference to the verb 'institute' does not have the same connotations as it might have in Anglo-American vernacular. As Andrew Goffey points out, in French, the term '*institution* does not cover the same semantic field as the English term "institution"' (Goffey, 2016: 39). Citing Jean Ayme on the history of institutional psychotherapy, Goffey reminds us that in French, '*institution* designates first of all the action of instituting, and then "everything that is invented by humans in opposition to the facts of nature"' (Ayme in Goffey, 2016: 39). What Anglophones might think of in relation to institutions is captured in French by the term 'establishment' (*établissement*). Citing Jean Oury, the founder of La Borde clinic where Guattari worked as a psychiatrist in the 1950s, Goffey makes a helpful distinction between institution and establishment which opens up the micropolitical potential of the transitional object as an institutional object:

> the establishment is a structure that is plunged into global society, and which relates to state criteria: it must answer to a large quantity of necessary administrative conditions; whereas *institutions* are something that can develop inside the establishment: they are quasi-infinite in number and variety. (Oury in Goffey, 2016: 39)

In Guattari's psychiatric practice, the therapy group at La Borde clinic acted as an institutional object whereby roles were examined and redistributed, the goal being to shift patients from dependency to autonomy. At La Borde, practical strategies involved the inclusion of everyone's interpretations in the group analysis as well as the allocation of duties such as cleaning and administration to doctors and patients. The purpose of this was to deterritorialize the hierarchical role of management which usually divides up those who need to be managed from those who manage, i.e. leaders. This idea can also be related to the Tavistock Method of group analysis which advocates curtailing the role of leader so as to enable group members to examine their intersubjective roles in the group. In fact, Ledare's interest in the Tavistock Method is that unlike a therapeutic model of analysis where the patient is dependent on the analyst, the role of leader or director is held off so that the group can explore their own roles.[10] In an article on the Tavistock Method of group relations in learning, E.R. Shapiro and A.W. Carr, while not using Guattarian terminology, nonetheless make the case that these groupings are about instituting their own institution as a microcosm that rethinks how work is shaped by the notion of the institution one carries in one's mind (2012: 78). Can it be said that the group dynamic in *The Large Group* produces something like a 'group-subject' that *institutes* itself and how might the viewer be incorporated into such a scene?

The male consultant, who sits in the inner circle surrounded by most of the group, advises them to get beyond the personal and to take the various provocations 'collectively'. He identifies two thematic strands from the group's tangential contributions, i.e. vulnerability and forgiveness, which might enable the group to manage the antagonisms that have broken out in this transitional space. Almost imperceptibly, as it is not reacted to immediately, this intervention seems to reorient the groups' attention towards questioning who is making the rules and what are the cultural conditions and constraints for action and speech. The consultants are accused of not providing leadership or guidance, a discussion that develops into group members concluding that there are two group mentalities, those who need a leader to galvanize them and those who believe people can self-organize. Strikingly their conclusions echo Bion's theory of groups and, while there is no resolution as such, the film gives a glimpse of the organizational knowledge that 'group-work mentality' can produce by distributing role-play across the group. A comment Ledare makes about his earlier work is apropos here in thinking about how subjectivation occurs by such means, what he refers to as 'a networked set of relations':

> How might a person in one position repurpose an asymmetry while someone else might utilize it in another way? How do these dynamics operate indirectly through triangulation for instance? And how might the intentions of any given gesture come to mean something different or be redefined inside a networked set of relations? Agency is a product of how subjects attune themselves to a specific context and how, tactically, they end up negotiating that structure. (Ledare in Kraus 2015: 60)

While the issue of how the cameras are mediating and perhaps producing behaviour is continually returned to by individual group members, mostly their presence is deemed unobtrusive. But what about the viewer? In order to follow the outbursts of tension that erupt and are managed transversally by group members, the viewer finds themselves moving almost like a camera as their gaze is directed to shift from one person to another, a movement reliant on the edit, which largely follows the sequence of the improvised conversation. In this, Ledare acts like the viewer's on-screen proxy, occasional cuts showing him intently following the to-and-fro between speakers. Addressed in this way, a viewer may identify with or recognize, judge and/or distance themselves from the behaviours and gestures performed by and in this assembly. But as a staged public clinic, which captures the 'microtemporal' gestures that operate beneath consciousness, the film might also serve as a transitional space enabling a viewer to test out their own issues of control and resistance without damaging consequences. In facilitating the potential of 'group-work mentality' to mitigate, without denying, the toxic effects of projection and prejudice, the film could be said to be inadvertently pedagogical without being moralistic.

The tensions and conflicts involved in interpersonal relations increase in Ledare's *The Task* which was filmed at The School of the Art Institute of Chicago for his exhibition in its gallery entitled 'The Plot'. As well as the film, 'The Plot' included vitrines of supporting material contextualizing the film. While also based on the Tavistock Institute's method of group analysis, *The Task* differs from *The Large Group* in being composed of an offshoot group, organized by Ledare, of a three-day Tavistock Group Relations Conference that was being held in Chicago.[11] Twenty-eight participants were included in the film as well as three consultants, six camera operators and three observers as well as Ledare. Ten psychologists also took part in the project. *The Task*, an 118-minute documentary, comprises seven chapters with intertitles such as 'Pre-Existing Conditions', 'Evictions' and 'Immune System' that document aspects of the last three of four group sessions that took place. Although the film is edited down to two hours from three and a half hours of footage, Ledare's intention was to retain the integrity and durational flow of the conversation. In some senses, *The Task* is less satisfying than *The Large Group*, though it is also more challenging. Representing a cross-section of the city's population, the racial, ethnic, gender and class tensions in *The Task* prevent anything like Bion's 'group-work mentality' from coming to the fore. In this sense, *The Task* is perhaps less politically optimistic than *The Large Group* as the group cannot be said to *institute* themselves per se. Nonetheless, in its ambition to assemble people who would not ordinarily encounter one another or attend Tavistock conferences, *The Task* does more than merely mirror social tensions, but tries to work through, rather than heal, them via the interface of group performance-to-camera. Ledare has said that he chose to 'shoot *The Task* in Chicago as an intervention, a kind of counter to the essentialism of what is still one of the most sharply segregated American cities'.[12] Rather than illumination, he was interested in Bion's notion of projecting 'a penetrating beam of darkness; a reciprocal of the searchlight' (Bion, 1990: 20) in order to engender 'an emergent lack of fixity, dynamics only ever being able to be seen indirectly [...] by way of contingency and triangulation'.[13] This motif of the searchlight echoes the microtemporal microanalysis that was enabled by the projected image in the therapeutic frameworks I referred to earlier.

In one of the sessions, Brad, a vocal middle-aged man sporting a ponytail, takes up a central seat in front of the older black male consultant, a gesture which is vociferously and literally interpreted by a red-haired white middle-aged artist who professes a particular interest in and knowledge of psychology. She makes no bones about explaining Brad's gesture as an unconscious desire to demand recognition from the consultant, Brad having previously confessed to being sexually assaulted by a black male babysitter when he was a child. A black woman adds to the interpretation by situating Brad's action as a way of regaining power over his previous trauma. There is no overt affirmation or refusal of this interpretation, the montage showing the exchange of looks between various participants across the visual field, a traversal that seems to hold a dichotomy of meanings in tandem without affirming any of them.

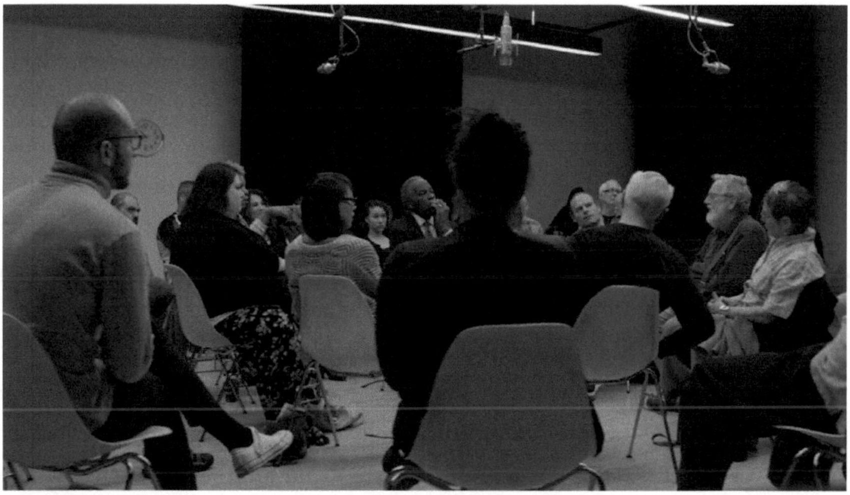

Figure 7.3 Leigh Ledare *The Task*, 2017. Courtesy of the artist.

Perhaps the 'interpretation' is plausible, perhaps it is too crude to be of value or perhaps it is a moment akin to Stiegler's 'Phew! It's out. Our sickness has been articulated', but rather than deciding once and for all what is true or false, the relay of roles in the group enables things to be said that, regardless of their truth, are effective in iterating what normally goes unsaid for fear of retribution or retaliation. And in so doing, prejudices and frustrations are voiced and heard without blame being attributed to individual protagonists. In this sense then, a modicum of 'group-work mentality' rises to the surface, although it disappears again into the individual issues of rejection and demands to be heard.

However, whereas in *The Large Group* Ledare honoured his contract with participants that his role would be purely observational, towards the end of *The Task* he felt impelled to violate that contract and intervene by joining the group's inner circle. The reason he gives for this in the film is to redirect the group's attention to the camera and the film crew as determinates of the situation. His intervention is perceived as a betrayal and an attack that results in the consultants, and the two group members experienced in the Tavistock Method, exiting the room in protest. The black male consultant summarizes his feelings to Ledare's intervention in terms of having had his 'balls [...] taken away'. This statement is revealing in that this consultant, true to the Tavistock Method of withholding the role of leader in the group, previously only intervened to divert the conversation away from the personal. His outburst exposes that this restraint was clearly his mode of enacting power in the group, his eruption leading to the group further fracturing and momentarily exacerbating the toxicities that were being held in the balance of its dynamic.

However, Ledare had other reasons for his intervention. It also stemmed from problems behind the scenes in that the conference director, who does not appear in the film, had tried to keep him off-side during the filming process and to stop the film from being completed.[14] Added to this, Ledare also claims that during the filming the psychologists created an in-group and an out-group between participants who had had experience of previous Tavistock conferences and those who did not. These 'group pairings' prevented the materialization of Ledare's intention which was for the group to consider 'the power structures that govern our relations to one another in a society where we are increasingly both observers and observed'.[15] While most participants considered Ledare's intrusion as a violation of his contract, on the other hand, a few were willing to take it 'collectively', implying that perhaps a future session might have redistributed the toxic defence mechanisms unleashed by his intervention. In Winnicottian terms, Ledare's intrusion could be viewed as a pre-emption of using the transitional object before the mediation between reality and fantasy had come to its own conclusion. In terms of the transitional object as institutional object, this would forestall the possibility of the group to *institute* itself. There are echoes here of Stiegler's critique of technics, i.e. that in the service of consumer capital, it short-circuits the infant's desire and demolishes the temporality required for adequate care to be provided by what Winnicott calls the environmental-mother.[16] For Stiegler, the mother's 'knowledge of the extra-ordinary character of the object' (2013a: 2), i.e. its pharmacological or conflictual nature, is upheld in the mother–child relation of transitional space, whereas, as I have already outlined, for Stiegler this upholding is being destroyed by the marketization that denies the conflictual nature of the object in favour of the immediate gratification of desire (2013a: 127). Rather than maintaining the pharmacological nature of the object as both poison and remedy, a process Stiegler calls adoption, this short-circuiting of desire moves the infant in the direction of an adaptation to the toxic (consumer) object. Applying this narrative to the social environment, adaptation thereby also extends to the ready acceptance of governance from the outside, the adaptive subject becoming more susceptible to an unquestioning reliance on others, political leaders for example, projecting the burden of its own toxicity onto them.

Reviewing *The Task* in the *Chicago Tribune*, Lori Waxman situates it in terms of contemporary communication in which privacy and intimacy are unrelentingly public, saying: 'It's reality television and social media, where performance and lived life are inextricably intertwined and available for manipulation. It's everything that's wrong with the world today, and yet we can't stop watching, commenting and posting' (2017). However, as I suggested in my preamble to this case study, the camera does not simply record a scene, but projects it, thereby revealing the subliminal interactions between participants that would otherwise be invisible to themselves as well as to viewers who might (dis)identify with them. Ledare refers to the situation as a learning experience that it is up to each group member, and perhaps the viewer, to metabolize for themselves. When *The Task* was exhibited at The Art Institute of Chicago in 2017, participants returned again and again to see themselves on-screen. I suggest that this has less to do with a commonsense notion of narcissism than with the fascination of being able to view how they operate as 'objects' for one another in the visual field, a view which is foreclosed on in everyday life. We can intuit how we are operating in the visual field, but recording devices transform this sensory vagueness into an object that might be 'used' in the Winnicottian sense. While the *institutional* organization of interpersonal relations in *The Task* is somewhat pre-empted by the various factors I've outlined, *The Large Group* takes this organization into itself.

In *The Large Group* this is represented by a drawing on the blackboard in the background, referred to as an organigram by one of the group members towards the end of the film. An organigram is a diagram that articulates the structure of an organization, which in this case appears as a fluid set of interweaving circles. In questioning its own organizational structure, the group could be said to be taking responsibility for its own relation to the 'infinite' or what Guattari refers to as the internal conflictual existence that groups often defend themselves against by uniting together in a common cause that enables them to project that conflict outside of themselves. For Guattari, as for Bion, there are two types of groups: subjugated groups and subject-groups. Subjugated groups come together to defend themselves against what they perceive as the threat of the outside. The group withdraws into itself by means of 'leaderships, identifications, effects of suggestion, disavowals, scape-goating, and so forth' (Guattari, 2015: 77). A subjugated group 'is a kind of syndicate or lobby of mutual defence against solitude, and of anything that might be classified as having a transcendental nature' (Guattari, 2015: 78). As opposed to this, what Guattari calls subject-groups are open-structures that are set up to dialogue outside of themselves. In order to do this, they have to internally take responsibility for the inherent human desire to project threat to the outside. Dealing with this desire from within can sometimes lead the group to implode. Subject-groups risk falling into chaos or, as Guattari says, 'being submerged in a flood of problems, tensions, internal battles, and risk of secession [...] thus develops a kind of vertigo, or madness peculiar to this group' (2015: 78). While Guattari's micropolitics is associated with subject-groups rather than subjugated groups, he maintains that a balance between these two tendencies is necessary.

However, in concluding this chapter, I am less concerned with evaluating whether and at what moments the groups in Ledare's films might become a subject-group than in considering them as pharmacological aesthetic objects. In a more speculative vein than the overtly therapeutic orientation of the image in my introductory vignettes, Guattari also proposed that films can operate as therapeutic modalities as they transport us to a guilt-free universe in which a film's 'semiotic components [...] glide by each other without fixing or stabilizing themselves' (Guattari, 2009: 263). While film is not immune from the modalities of repressive power, for Guattari its

> asignifying semiotic chains of intensities, movements, and multiplicities fundamentally tends to free it from the signifying grid that intervenes only at a second stage, through the filmic syntagmatic that fixes genres, crystallizes characters and behavioural stereotypes homogeneous to the dominant semantic field. (263)

For Guattari, the effects of 'desubjectivation and deindividuation produced by the *énoncé* in cinema or in such arrangements as drugs, dreaming, passion, creation, delirium, etc.' (2009: 262) are bound up with the cinematic affects of colour and sound beyond or outside of narrative rather than the kinds of discursive moving image artworks I am looking at here. However, in 'The Poor Man's Couch', he also links 'film-viewing' acts to speech acts, arguing that their performativity engenders a suspension of usual modes of communication unlike the reinforcement of dominant discourse in 'psychoanalytical performance' (2009: 258). Now while Guattari is not referring to discursive speech acts per se, I would nonetheless claim that, in Ledare's *The Large Group*, something like Guattari's 'group-subject' occurs in which the group *institute* a space in which their need to control and judge is suspended and a facility to analyse and enact roles in a more playful, less rigid, way emerges. Their initial free association from 'Leigh' to 'wine' alludes to this. As a pharmacological moving image artwork, *The Large Group* plays with the controls of readymade discourses – of therapy, of surveillance – and, in so doing, these discourses become micropolitical acts of organizational *instituting* (my emphasis), albeit in a staged setting. In this, the pharmacological therapeutics of his films could be said to provide a model of how 'group-mentality work' might alleviate subjection and engender the 'feed-forward structure' of subjectivation. Guattari would undoubtedly consider Ledare's work as part of the discursive narrativity he claims as subjugating and against which he opposes the asignifying 'traits of matter of expression of other components [...] plastic, spatial or musical materials' (Guattari, 2011: 47).[17] However, I claim that the discursive performativity of moving image artworks such as *The Large Group* and those by the contemporary women artists I shall examine in the next three chapters opens up a space of self- or group-*instituting* beyond the supposed subjection to dominant signifying semiologies, i.e. stereotypical and categorical identities. In facilitating the performance of the latter as objects to be tested and played with under the 'objectifying eye of the camera', Ledare's pharmacological aesthetics straddles both poison and cure.

8

Aesthetic modes of performative truth-telling in *The O Show* and *Self Made*

In this chapter I shall further explore the pharmacological therapeutic aesthetics of self-authoring in relation to works by two artists: Oriana Fox and Gillian Wearing. In both case studies, this occurs through performative truth-telling. Performative truth-telling is not the same as the impetus to tell the truth which, in common parlance as well as in philosophy, implies an ideal that in practice is necessarily compromised. We can recall Stiegler's notion that anamnesis, i.e. the act of memory which for Plato is linked to truth-telling, is predicated on hypomnesis, i.e. technologies of recording. Thereby, truth-telling is always in the process of being transduced through a medium rather than issuing from an essential separable self. The notion of truth as a performative modality that straddles the fictional and the real cogently emerges in the conversations between psychoanalyst Arabella Kurtz and novelist J.M. Coetzee in *The Good Story: Exchanges on Truth, Fiction and Psychoanalytic Psychotherapy* (2015). Over the course of their conversations, therapeutic discourse becomes connected to fiction and/or performativity as a mode of productive, rather than curative, truth-telling. As this notion is key to my discussion of Fox and Wearing in what follows, I want to précis it here.

Coetzee, who has never been in analysis, raises the question of fictional truth in contrast to Kurtz's insistence on the discovery of an 'internal truth' (11), which is, for her, the goal of psychoanalytic therapy. As opposed to the singularity of Kurtz's 'internal truth', for Coetzee the ethics of living involves giving an account of oneself in which fictional truths co-exist. These two views may seem far removed from one another; however, what develops in their conversations is the notion that both forms of 'truth' are constructions of sorts.

All life-narratives are constructions in the sense of shaping and structuring what would otherwise be sensory fragments and intangible imprinted memories. Coetzee questions Kurtz:

> What is it that impels you, as a therapist, to want your patient to confront the truth about themself, as opposed to collaborating or colluding in a story – let us call it a fiction, but an empowering fiction – that would make the patient feel good about themself, good enough to go out into the world better able to love and work? (3)

While Coetzee's idea of there being 'versions of the truth' (6) initially seems at odds with Kurtz's finding of an internal 'emotional truth' (9), links between them emerge. Kurtz admits that in the case of the latter:

> It is not that some fixed and external truth exists and is gradually and painstakingly accessed [. . .] the truth in psychotherapy is in its essence dynamic because it derives from the perspective of a living being whose external and internal characteristics change, even in small ways, over time. (10)

Thereby Coetzee's notion that a life-story is 'a compendium of memories which one is free to interpret in the present according to the demands (and desires) of the present' (13) is not unrelated to Kurtz's analytic situation in which truth is relational and emergent. As she says: 'an I-and-you truth is much more valuable than one more separate and more certain' (137). This truth can be said to be pharmacological. It is not a transcendental truth but an ongoing process of being able to tolerate the painful uncertainty that one cannot know the truth.[1]

Relational truths circulate in Fox's *The O Show* (2011–ongoing), episodes of which are performed live for an (art) audience with edited videos distributed online[2] and Wearing's experimental documentary *Self Made* (2010). Both works could be said to manufacture their truth-effects through the performance of on-screen life-narratives and both works deploy therapeutic techniques to enact these performances: respectively, Rational emotive behaviour therapy (REBT), a form of therapy invented in the mid-1950s by Dr Albert Ellis, and Method, an acting technique developed in the early twentieth century by the Russian theatre director and actor Konstantin Stanislavski. Both works propose the repair of damaged or toxic selves, but they also raise questions about their own toxicity as media forms dependent on performative speech, in both the theatrical and the linguistic sense (Parker and Sedgwick, 1995).[3] REBT is explicitly referred to on Episode 3 of Fox's *The O Show* (2012), one of her three guests being her real-life REBT therapist Bernadette Ainsworth. As opposed to Ainsworth's bio-psychosocial model of emotional disturbance or trauma that may be remedied in as little as a couple of sessions, the other two guests – a psychodynamic therapist, Liz Bentley, and Method acting coach, Sam Rumbelow, who also features in *Self Made* – refer to the extended temporality of 'sitting with an emotion' in contrast to the quick fix of REBT. However, there are uncanny parallels between both these therapeutic techniques that neatly align with governmental exhortations to well-being and health, in the UK at least. Both techniques, especially the cognitive behavioural therapies (CBTs), of which REBT is one, are more cost effective than the longer-term investment in the psychoanalytic talking cure. CBT in particular is deemed efficient in providing fast 'cures' that enable more productive citizens, which is why it is recommended as a treatment for work-related depression, including unemployment. In an era of cognitive capitalism, not only is the production of autonomous well-adapted behavioural selves and psyches desirable, regardless of one's social and economic circumstances, but emotional and cognitive reorientation is also deemed possible. CBT is considered an efficient remedy to heal the anxieties that ensue from social, economic and technological change, as the therapy advocates changing individual thinking about one's circumstances rather than challenging the social conditions that might be causing one's problems in the first place.[4] That said, in this chapter, I will nonetheless extend my pharmacological approach from simply being a diagnosis that exposes symptoms to explore how on-screen performances might be therapeutically 'curative' in ways that skirt close to the prevailing discourses in cognitive capitalism that values aspirational subjects unhindered by trauma. My homeopathic mimetic approach has affinity with Fox's description of her methods as looking like they are promoting aspirational subjectivities that align with neoliberal cognitive capitalist values of success and achievement, but that they are undertaken for different ethical reasons and this makes all the difference.[5] So while my examples may seem somewhat counterintuitive in that they can be read as proffering feel-good versions of selfhood, my argument will be that they nonetheless complicate the promise of cure without, however, foreclosing on its potential for personal transformation.

Appearing to be operating within the parameters of neoliberal values, they reorient these values towards non-normative ends.[6]

Fox's *The O Show* reprises her interest in televisual media narratives of self-improvement in her videos such as *Our Bodies, Ourselves* (2003) and her remake of the TV series *Sex and the City* (2003), in which she acted the roles of all four female characters, mashing the consumerist romantic narrative of the TV series with second-wave feminist art. Rather than purchasing the latest designer style, her characters sat around sewing vaginal imagery on quilts and such like. Historically, artistic mediums such as needlework and embroidery signified female emancipation and autonomy both for the suffragettes and for leading artists of second-wave feminist art such as Judy Chicago. However, in the contemporary climate of neoliberal capitalism, the ideals of female autonomy that characterized the Women's Liberation Movement have been compromised by their proximity to the goals of consumer capital. As Catherine Rottenberg argues, in the entanglement of feminist progressivist politics with neoliberalism, words such as 'equal rights, liberation and social justice' which traditionally formed the basis of feminist public debates and discussions have been somewhat overtaken by words such as 'happiness, balance, responsibility and lean in' (2018: 5). Acquiring such 'goods' increases a woman's social capital in a context that 'recasts individuals as capital-enhancing agents' (Rottenberg, 2018: 7). As we shall see in Fox's work, therapeutic techniques can be used as a means of acquiring and managing these goods. However, this is not to say that they cannot be reoriented to other uncommodified ends such as the necessity of an aesthetics of everyday survival in the face of the 'bulldozer' concepts such as neoliberalism (and, to a lesser degree, cognitive capitalism) that act as incapacitating metanarratives. For Fox, *The O Show* is about the therapeutic potential of performance and the first episode's guests include performance artists for whom 'acting out' their fears and anxieties has an empowering dimension.[7] However, I want to focus on two episodes: Episode 3: The Therapeutic Potential of Performance (2012) and Episode 8: You're Only as Sick as Your Secrets (2018). Episode 3 allows me to continue with a pharmacological critique of the therapeutic while Episode 8 enables me to move towards a more 'curative' set of truth-effects, undoubtedly influenced by my having attended its live iteration and witnessing the Q&A that is not included in the edited online video.

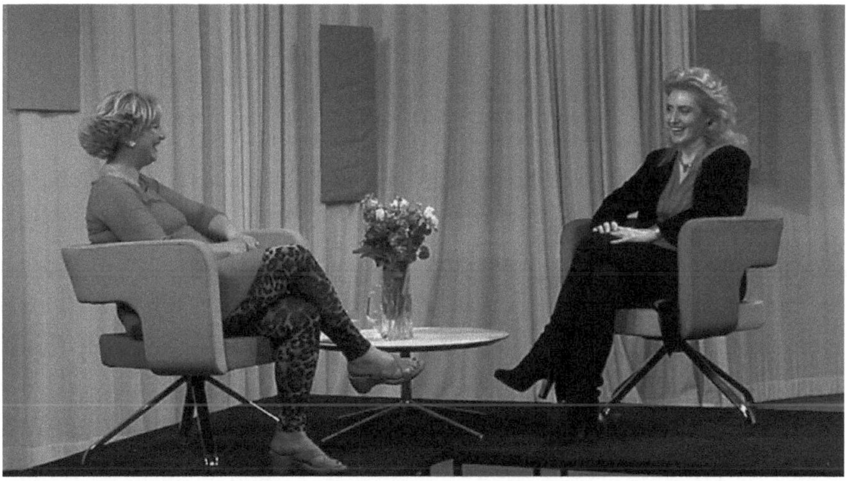

Figure 8.1 Oriana Fox, *The O Show: The Therapeutic Potential of Performance*, 2012. (video still) Courtesy of the artist.

As I have said, Episode 3 features Fox interviewing her REBT therapist, Bernadette Ainsworth, who previously worked as an actress and is a persuasive advocate of REBT. She charismatically professes that the therapy transforms people for the better, solving personal anxieties and emotional disturbances more successfully than other therapies such as psychoanalysis which is unnecessarily time consuming and expensive. The premise of REBT is taking emotional responsibility for how one thinks and feels about situations, in other words, a crude performativity dependent on a volitional subject in control of its destiny rather than being subject to what Butler calls the 'constitutive constraints' of body and psyche (1993: 96). Without any apparent irony, Ainsworth breezily aligns REBT's ethos of choosing the kind of emotional life you want to have with consumerist capitalist society, saying that the success of REBT is its capacity to achieve 'fast, efficient and speedy results'. Fox, Ainsworth states, is living proof of this, as, after trying various psychoanalytic and psychodynamic therapies, REBT was the therapy that finally worked. 'That *is* the narrative!' Fox retorts ironically as if to throw its validity into doubt, though the camera's deliberate gaze on Fox's pregnant belly seems to further underscore Ainsworth's success in enabling Fox's achievements. Fox appears as both glamorous faux-TV host, successful artist and a future mother, all roles endorsed as fulfilling the social contract to be re/productive as well as linking to neoliberal feminism's notion that a woman can have it all, sometimes referred to as 'lean in' feminism.[8]

Fox blogs that 'the techniques illuminated by these professionals can be employed towards achieving ever increasing happiness, self-actualization and creative productivity'.[9] The statement sardonically mirrors current governmental edicts on well-being in the UK. Not only is it socially desirable, but creative activities are deemed instrumental to its achievement. The population at large are exhorted to engage in such activities, not only improve the happiness index, but to partake in the good life that is available to all if only they would choose it rather than damaging themselves in self-induced psychopathologies and addictions. This exhortation is made without paying adequate attention to major shifts in infrastructure, such as lack of funding and investment, that disable access to such creative activities. It emphasizes individual responsibility for well-being, as well as social prescribing by general practitioners and others working in the welfare system. Situated in relation to this context, Fox's show could be said to be platforming a technique that potentially could be used by everyone to efficiently and quickly reduce the pathologies that stem from what Han calls 'achievement society' (2015: 8). Her show could be said to evidence the commodification of emotions endemic to a cognitive capitalist economy in which the transformation of negative feelings into positive attitudes enables the acquisition of social capital that can be exchanged in competitive labour markets, including the art world. Fox introduces episodes of *The O Show* by telling her own story of successful recovery, how she used REBT to gain control over problems that inhibited productive functioning in everyday life, mainly severe shyness. Her invited guests have usually overcome or managed various emotional and/or mental health issues through practicing some form of therapeutic technique. They often exude the affirmative positivity of post-trauma survival that is exhibited on reality TV shows and lapped up by audiences who themselves may be aspirational subjects suffering from the fallout of 'achievement society' which Han characterizes as being beset with '[n]eurological illnesses such as depression, attention deficit hyperactivity disorder (ADHD), borderline personality disorder (BPD), and burnout syndrome' (2015: 1). Han sees these pathologies as stemming from 'the excess of positivity' that pervades a contemporary social and technological landscape in which negativity is banished (4). REBT's advocacy of positivity could be said to be a form of psychic entrepreneurialism.

Shame-attacking, which Fox advocates on her show, is key to this positivity. This technique promotes an approach to personal problems in which a 'client', moving towards the total self-acceptance advocated by REBT, deliberately acts out in ways they fear might incite judgement from others. Fox calls this 'acting against one's irrational beliefs'; Ainsworth refers to it as 'exposure and response prevention'.[10] Surviving the act, a person realizes that no one is judging them and that nothing bad happens if they act out what they desire to become. In Fox's case, this entailed the repeated pretence of being confident to enable her to actually become more confident and be cured of shyness, a kind of 'fake it till you make it' production of identity.[11] The performative iteration of the speech-act 'I am confident' produces a 'truth-effect' or an 'empowering fiction' as Coetzee referred to it above.[12] Rather than adhering to a notion of truth as fixed in the past, e.g. 'I am shy and nothing will change that', the speech act engenders a 'fictional truth' that comes from the future to empower a present that will, in the process, become that future. This kind of artistic practice is not unique to Fox.

While not referring to REBT, the artist Ann Hirsch describes her YouTube performances as the character Caroline Benton on her vlog *Scandalishious* (2010) as a form of 'exposure therapy'.[13] Benton is a twenty-something hipster with a squeaky cloying voice who performs song and dance routines for her followers as well as confessing her anxieties and desires. Hirsch's discussion of this fits with the therapeutic narrative of self-esteem that Fox deploys in her chat show:

> While I was growing up and becoming a woman, I hated myself. I knew I was smart but other than that I thought I was just a disgusting girl that no one could be sexually interested in. I started performing as *Scandalishious* because I was tired of feeling that way. Or at least, I was tired of appearing as though I felt that way. So I started pretending I thought I was sexy and I quickly learned that if I pretended to be confident, people would believe it. And then I actually became more confident as a result. (Hirsch in Archey, 2012)

While on the one hand this persona enables Hirsch to mimic the narcissism of online female subjectivities, it is also a vehicle to express and work on her own feelings of insecurity and shame around sexuality.[14] Hirsch could be said to use her Caroline character to act against irrational beliefs that in the philosophy of REBT are seen as stemming from subconscious core ideas and attachment to 'underlying "rules" about how the world and life should be' (Froggatt, 2005). While the misogyny that Hirsch purports to have unconsciously imbibed does exist, her decision to act against how that phenomenon affected her resonates with REBT which advocates moving away from applying general traits and external judgements to rate the 'self'.

The use of 'exposure therapy' as a way of producing 'truth-effects' is very different from the therapeutic proclaiming of one's truth in art discourse of the 1990s. Early in the decade, art historian Hal Foster was critical of confessional art by artists such as Sue Williams and of reality TV chat shows for naturalizing damaged, victimized and traumatized bodies as an ur-ground of authentic experience (Foster, 1996a). His reasoning was that this recourse to personal trauma makes experience impossible to challenge or criticize as the subject proffers their truth as irrefutable. By contrast, in Foster's poststructuralist approach to subjectivity, the subject is split from knowing itself, whereas to proclaim the truth of a unified self disavows the internal opacity of the subject, thereby risking the danger of projecting it outwards in unwitting acts of domination and/or the phobic exclusion of others.[15] In Foster's art world milieu, however, the incursion of the confessional subject into art, which he considered problematic, also had political import. Echoing earlier 1970s feminist art in which the confessional was intrinsic to a critique of patriarchal injunctions to repress the personal voices of women, the identity politics of the 1990s promulgated the albeit traumatized identity of the self as the essential ground from which to demand political transformation. However, this injunction to speak one's trauma has today transformed into a desirable form of micro-celebrity in which everyone can be an actor or protagonist in their own drama, a form of public display which segues with the neoliberal impetus to aspirational selfhood in a competitive cycle of self-improvement.

As Furedi recounts it, the idiom of therapeutics to describe the self spiralled in the 1990s, its initial emphasis on trauma as a particular overwhelming form of experience gradually transforming by the end of the decade to become a figure of speech referring to little more than people's response to an unpleasant situation (2004: 4). His polemical view is somewhat echoed by Illouz in her analysis of how therapeutic communication in cognitive capitalism instils a procedural quality to emotional life in which emotions are subject to measurement (2007). In this development, emotions become divorced from their fluctuating situational contexts and more compatible with 'a language of rights and of economic productivity' (Illouz, 2007: 38). In this shift, negative emotions such as guilt, anger, resentment, shame or frustration are neutralized in the subjection of emotional relationships to management procedures. While on the one hand, REBT's technique of shame-attacking, in enabling people to overcome their fears by acting them out, seems laudable, it also appears to tally with the underlying tenet in neoliberal cognitive capitalism that we have both the right to and the responsibility for our own well-being and happiness. The inability to take control of this is seen as personal failure rather than stemming from wider systemic issues. For Illouz, in earlier forms of capitalism the 'subject could shift back and forth from the "strategic" to the purely "emotional"' (2007: 110), as the public and the private spheres of life were kept separate. However, in an era of psychology and the internet in which therapeutic emotional styles are ubiquitous, the contemporary subject of capitalism is 'increasingly split between a hyperrationality which has commodified and rationalized the self, and a private world increasingly dominated by self-generated fantasies' (Illouz, 2007: 113). On the other hand, the evolution of the private sphere into a social declamatory-space in contemporary media such as *The O Show* and *Scandalishious* somewhat overrules Illouz's split between public and private and may signal a means by which something genuine and transformative might emerge.[16]

What I am getting at here is alluded to in Rob Horning's discussion of performative truth-telling in his online essay 'Games of Truth' (2013) which, although specific to social media, is of interest here in relation to Hirsch's and Fox's forms of 'exposure therapy'. For Horning, critics of social media's supposed inauthenticity mistake it as performance or 'strategic' playacting, but he insists, citing Wayne Koestenbaum, that it can be a way of re-inscribing authenticity in a world that seems increasingly to be filled with fakeness. Key to his argument is that 'as more behavior seems inauthentic and performative, there is a greater need to expose ourselves and have our own authenticity vindicated through the embarrassment this causes us' (Horning, 2013). Horning aligns this method of exposure (therapy) to the figure of the cynic as discussed by Foucault in his last two lecture series at the Collège de France in 1982–83 and 1983–84, respectively published in English as *The Government of Self and Others* and *The Courage of the Truth*. The cynic in ancient Greece is the one who speaks the truth to the king, exposing as lies, what masquerades as truth. Foucault refers to the cynic's performance of truth-telling as a form of parrhesia or free speech, a plain-speaking truth marked by provocation in which the truth content of an utterance is indexed to the risk that might be incurred in speaking it. As Sergei Prozorov states, for the cynics, 'truth-telling is only possible as an act of disobedience in the face of all social norms and conventions' (2017).[17] But this act of disobedience is not oppositional. Rather it reclaims one's power from the social order and its rationalities of government by living with and applying it to oneself in a subjectivation, i.e. a self-forming practice, that transvalues the biopolitical attempt to impose order on the self. (For me, this transvaluation is reminiscent of the strategy of homeopathic mimicry which I shall return to towards the end of this chapter.) As Prozorov states:

> The parrhesiast does not resist governmental biopower but demonstrates in its very practice of the true life how it has always already failed to transform and govern one's life, while s/he has on the contrary succeeded in doing so by reclaiming its own biopower and applying it to oneself. (2017)

Therein lies an oblique connection to shame-attacking and, in fact, Foucault's use of parrhesia is also one of Fox's main theoretical inspirations, enabling her to avoid 'seeking out some essential truth at the core of [...] identity'.[18] Acting as if she is confident allows her to become 'someone I never thought I could be. I am also able to tell truths in this way without limiting my sense of myself to a single and limiting truth'.[19]

While it may be a bit of a leap to connect the ancient Greek speech-act of parrhesia to shame-attacking,[20] the performing of shameful acts in the latter resonates with the cynic's beastly antics in speaking the truth to power as a means of empowerment. Apposite here is Foucault's account of the shift in the 'parrhesiastic game' from the classical Greek conception, in which the cynic courageously speaks the truth to the king, to 'another truth game which now consists in being courageous enough to disclose the truth about oneself' (Foucault in Pearson, 1985: 55). This new kind of 'parrhesiastic game' requires practical training or exercises that are 'concerned with endowing the individual with the preparation and the moral equipment that will permit him to fully confront the world in an ethical and rational manner' (Foucault in

Pearson, 1985: 58). Although the training developed by the cynics in ancient Greece involves a much more long-term practice of self-scrutiny than that advocated in REBT, Fox's use of the therapy in her performative art practice enables social behaviours that produce self-actualization without necessarily adapting to the status quo.

In 'Therapy for a Pathological Capitalism' (2014), Karl Lydén also refers to Foucault's analysis of parrhesia as obliquely offering a model of therapy in cognitive capitalism. Lydén identifies the conditions of the latter as a three-headed hydra in which social subjects could be simultaneously:

> employed, perhaps, in the sector of manufacture or in any case forming part of abstract labor, and – whether it is during work time or leisure time – consuming and producing value within the social realm, while having to deal with an increasingly deplete, slow, hostile, and rigid state apparatus in order to receive basic social functions like health care, education, and unemployment benefits when needed. (2014: 118)

Posing the question of what the therapy for the pathologies generated by such conditions might be, he too turns to Foucault's aforementioned lectures in which he addresses care of the self.[21] Exploring how 'subjects could constitute themselves in care of the self, consisting in acts and practices of truth' (2014: 119), Lydén focuses on Foucault's discussion of a particular obscure community called the Therapeutae who lived in small suburban gardens outside Alexandria in Ancient Greece. Group members retreated to this area, in which each had their own cell with some communal areas, in order to cure both spiritual and physical illness by mastering the self and caring for the body using exercises such as fasting and meditation. In his interest in these practices, Foucault passes from a theory of the subject 'to the analysis of the modalities and techniques of the relation to self' (Lydén, 2014: 121). Rather than this being a purely individualistic exercise, this ancient religious community maintained the competency of all individuals regardless of class or wielding of political power to be 'able to carry out this practice of the self' (Foucault in Lydén, 2014: 124). For Lydén, its social dimension consists in

> the collective shaping of a communist set of practices, cares, and acts of truth as the cures for our most acute pathologies. That is to say, one would have to withdraw together with others and form separate communities, whether it

> is in small suburban gardens like the *Therapeutae* or in other places, in order to embark on the collective care of the self and others. (129)[22]

Fox's chat show project, while not a retreat into seclusion, nonetheless advocates social competency, Fox promoting shame-attacking as a technique that anyone can deploy in their lives, while her guests have usually found other popular and often communal therapeutic modes and techniques of behaviour that afford them the license and confidence to become themselves. I have attended two of the filming sessions as a member of the public, the second of which, held at Block 336 gallery in London on 10 December 2018, was particularly interesting in terms of pharmacological aesthetics as involving both critical diagnosis and transformative potential. The live performance of this episode 'You're Only as Sick as Your Secrets' featured interviews with four guests who have publicly disclosed their own battles with mental health, namely: writer and activist Hamja Ahsan; circus performer Jess Love; writer and Lacanian psychoanalyst Anouchka Grose; and artist Kim Noble.

As befits live performance, the audience is not only given insight into aspects of behind-the-scenes production but participates in the process, Fox

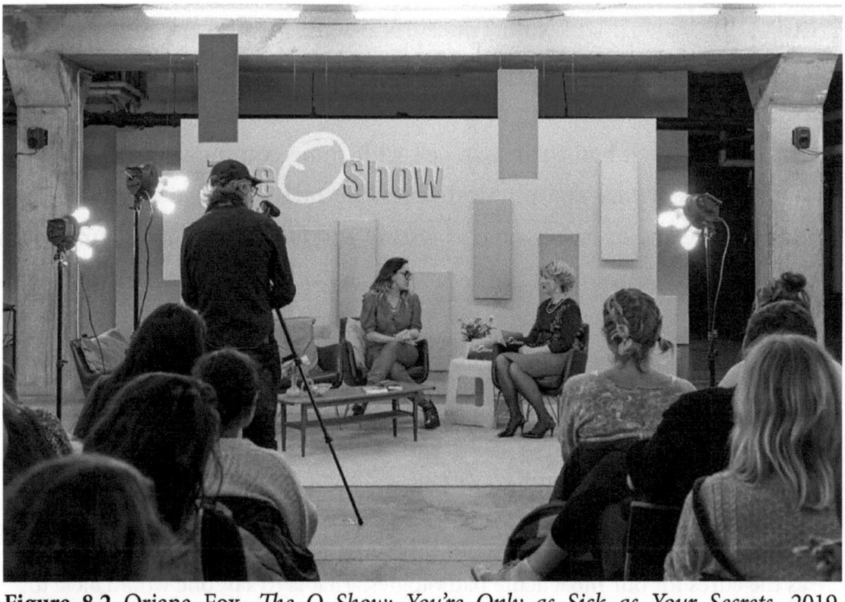

Figure 8.2 Oriana Fox, *The O Show: You're Only as Sick as Your Secrets*, 2019. (production still) Courtesy of the artist and Block 336.

giving instructions about when to laugh and how to respond to her opening lines. She also visibly directs the camera crew, deciding on retakes and asking them questions throughout about camera angles and views. Interviews are constantly being interrupted and reshot in the process. However, the exposure of the production process did not prevent the audience from identifying with the confessional ethos of *The O Show* to perform their own parrhesiastic speech-acts. In the Q&A following the interviews, audience members' personal contributions communicated to me that the millennial generation, representatives of which were the main respondents, may think differently about symptoms such as anxiety and depression than how these symptoms are classified by and dealt with in established institutions as being a deterrent to achievement. A general sense emerged from the predominantly young audience that, while medical diagnoses are extremely useful in accessing services and in giving a psychological disorder a shape, they themselves had more playful approaches to their 'symptoms' much as Fox does in her show. Of course, I am not suggesting that all mental health disorders can be played with, but within the range of disorders that this audience presented to one another in the Q&A, e.g. anxiety, depression and certain forms of bipolar disorder, audience members (and guests) had a more humorous, ironic sense of their symptoms than that which is portrayed in official discourse. The encouragement to situate one's symptom in a more ambivalently playful ways was, I think, partly inspired by Ahsan's contribution to the discussion. While emphasizing the value of diagnosis, Ahsan also advocated the collective power and resistance of what he referred to as a healing silence as opposed to always rising to the injunction to speak from the place of one's 'trauma'. To do the latter supports a status quo that wants those it considers minorities to reify their trauma in identitarian terms. This enables 'them' to be treated to adapt rather than the symptom engendering a shift in how society organizes its classifications of health and illness. Ahsan asserted that his shyness is an integral part of himself that is neither reducible to his being categorized as neuro-atypical nor something that he wants to eradicate to fit in better with the assertive subjectivity promulgated in mainstream society. Rather than seeing Fox's use of REBT as being part of the management of emotional life that Illouz aligns with entrapment in cognitive capitalism, it can be viewed as reorienting the latter's injunction to achieve success by appropriating a mode of self-authorization and making it distinct from governmentality. The online videos of the show, rather than offering recipes for self-improvement, act like place holders for emotional work that goes on elsewhere, behind the scenes as it were, in the everyday live acts of their protagonists and audiences. In this sense, it could be said to have links with Wearing's 'fictional' documentary *Self Made*.[23]

Wearing describes *Self Made* as 'the search for authenticity in the dramatic moment, and the possibilities of creativity'.[24] Her first and only feature, the film reprises many elements of her multi-media art practice informed by an interest in reality TV and questions of documentary truth, especially the video installation *Confess All on video. Don't Worry. You Will Be in Disguise. Intrigued? Call Gillian* (1994). To cast the latter, Wearing placed an advertisement using the title of the proposed work in the magazine *Time Out*. For *Self Made,* she placed a similar ad in newspapers, job centres and online. The ad, which appears on-screen in the opening moments of the film, reads 'Would you like to be in a film? You can play yourself or a fictional character. Call Gillian.' Unlike *Confess All on video* in which the participants wear masks while recounting tales of trauma and abuse to an off-screen Wearing,[25] in *Self Made* the seven respondents appear as 'themselves', chosen, as their on- and off-screen method coach Rumbelow continually reminds them, because they had interesting stories to tell. All wanted to explore some emotionally disturbing dynamic in their lives to try and get a perspective on it, e.g. issues of abandonment, violence, bullying and the desire to commit suicide.

On one level *Self-Made* is a highly edited documentary about the Method-acting workshops undergone by its seven non-actor participants as training for their personal 'end films', five of which, straddling genres from theatre, TV and cinema, are included in the main film.[26] Underscoring its use of documentary conventions, the film includes a number of talking heads sequences in which the participants introduce themselves, and, more importantly, in which they comment on how they feel about their 'end films' after viewing them off-screen. Further exposing the constructed nature of the documentary (which to my mind is unnecessary in a media environment in which mainstream productions commonly use such supposed critical techniques), shots of the crew are inserted in a couple of sequences, one of which includes an appearance by Wearing directing a participant's 'end film'.

The film opens with the first part of participant Asheq Akhtar's 'end film', a sequence which is repeated in full towards the end of the film, but this time using different camera angles and positions, again drawing attention to the constructed nature of documentary editing. This makes *Self Made* sound as if its goal is to reveal the mechanics behind the artifice, an interpretation which would not only be reductive but would also be a limited approach to artists' filmmaking in a media ecology in which there is much cross-genre pollination and heightened audience media literacy. Such an interpretation would be an example of 'paranoid criticism', an approach that 'trust[s] in exposure' and misguidedly 'depends [...] on an infinite reservoir of naiveté in those who make up the audience for these unveilings' (Sedgwick, 2003: 141). In *Self Made*, Wearing does engage in minimal 'paranoid' acts of exposure, i.e. critical alienation, as if to comfort an art audience that their looking at others has the moral tenor of reflexivity. In fact, artist and theorist colleagues of mine view *Self Made* with scepticism, if not outright condemnation, for what they see as its manipulation of participants' traumatic experiences. The documentary aspect of Wearing's film is viewed as creating the problematic illusion that its art audience are privileged witnesses or voyeurs of others' re-enactments of traumatic experience using exercises and techniques usually deployed in the privacy of behind-the-scenes rehearsals or Method training classes. The unease at this potential voyeurism is accentuated by the fact that some of the film's participants, while volunteering to explore personal traumas on-screen, can be identified as being working-class and/or of immigrant descent. The website for *Self Made* contains numerous accolades but the negative responses to the film that I have encountered in my peer group echo the mixed reception by art audiences of Richard Billingham's early documentary-style film *Fishtank* (1998) portraying his drunken alcoholic father Ray and his mother Liz, an obese chain smoker, in their British Midlands tower block flat. For some critics, Billingham's film objectifies the working-class other for privileged art audiences, thereby feeding the desire for a voyeuristic a kind of poverty porn, mitigated in this case by the fact that the artist is portraying his own family rather than subjecting unknown others to his camera gaze as Wearing does in *Self Made*. British middle-class art audiences appear to me to have conflictual feelings of curiosity and shame when viewing people from working-class backgrounds, feeling uncomfortable about the danger of further objectifying those who are either vilified or nostalgically celebrated in mainstream media. However, this moral discomfort fails to attribute autonomy to the self-styling capacities of working-class people on-screen. By contrast to this misguided view, *Self Made* shows how Method can be used by anyone to both mine and liberate core beliefs and habits by imaginatively inventing situations whose 'truth-effects' can be played with rather than used to solidify a prescribed and proscriptive identity. In this, *Self Made* is also invested in the therapeutic potential of performance.

Method is a technique that trains actors to relate to their characters by finding a truth in themselves, a sense memory, which can be tapped into to embody said character. This sense memory can be used as a tool to create the paradox of authentic impersonations which propel action forwards in time rather than reasserting a truth of the past. This use of Method as a tool for the elaboration of 'truth-effects' is akin to the goal of shame-attacking in Fox's work with the proviso that here new impersonations are developed through 'sense-memory' rather than through 'plain-speaking'. In *Self Made*'s highly edited Method workshops, Rumbelow instructs participants to enter into imaginary scenarios and play with their sense memories to find what he advocates as their 'truth'. In this, the film recalls Coetzee's and Kurtz's discussion in which raiding the memory-store to rewrite the life-story rather than fixing memory in the past is considered productive of 'fictional truths' that may enable people to play more creatively with their lives (2015: 6).

This 'fictional truth' is tapped into using relaxation techniques and role-play, the workshops acting as a kind of safe space that facilitate the emergence of buried emotions, not as they were in the past – there is no analysis here – but as they might relate to the present task of generating transformative futures. Crucial to this transformative potential is the fact that the participants' 'end films' are self-invented narratives or scenes chosen by them in order to enact the fears and disappointments that they consider keep them locked in crippling mind-sets. In a workshop exploring the capacity to express anger, Rumbelow encourages one of the participants, Lesley, to confront, rather than hide, her sadness. In response to her reluctantly admitting feeling sad after smashing a load of crockery against the wall, his affirmation gives her permission to unashamedly use this emotion in her 'end film' in which she stars as a 1940s heroine who rejects the attentions of an admiring man rather

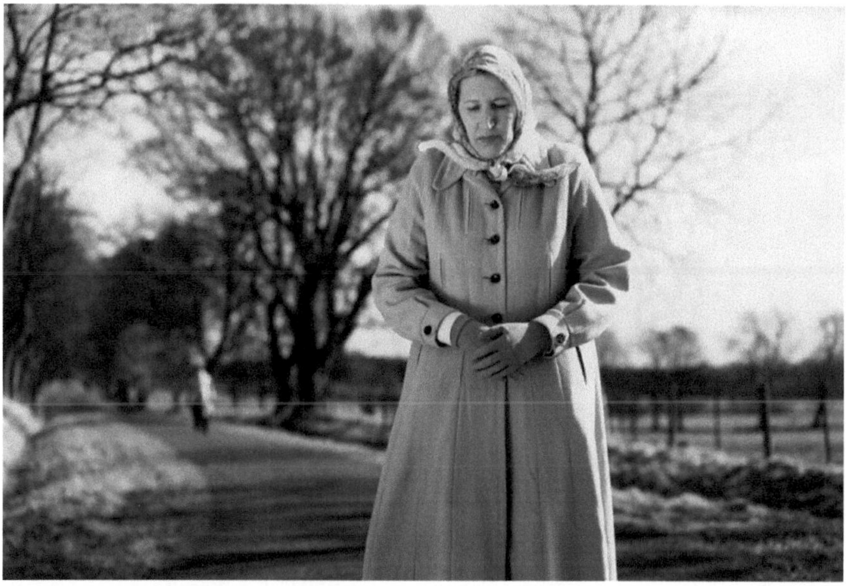

Figure 8.3 Gillian Wearing *Self Made* (2010) colour film with sound, 84 minutes. © Gillian Wearing, courtesy Maureen Paley, London.

than trust him, although she longs for companionship both in real life and in the film. The acting-out of this desire, akin to the impetus of shame-attacking, enables her to see its impact on her life. It does not transform her into a person who is not shy and distrustful but enables her to accept herself without judgement. That performative acting-out can have psychological effects on the individual, changing how they might behave in the future, is shown even more emphatically and disturbingly in relation to another participant, Asheq, or Ash as he is referred to in the film.

Ash breaks into tears at various points in the film. The editing of the film at these points, while not as aggressive as the probing camera work in mainstream documentaries such as those by Michael Moore or Nick Broomfield, nonetheless homes in on Ash as if hounding his character. Two scenes stand out here. In one of the workshops, Rumbelow directs the seven participants to visualize being immersed in tepid bathwater. They sway, eyes closed, on plastic chairs, making the kinds of guttural sounds, ah ah-ing and coughing, he previously instructed them to use as a technique of releasing emotion. The visualization brings Ash to his first breakdown. He starts to choke. It makes for uncomfortable viewing. Is this a glimpse of something

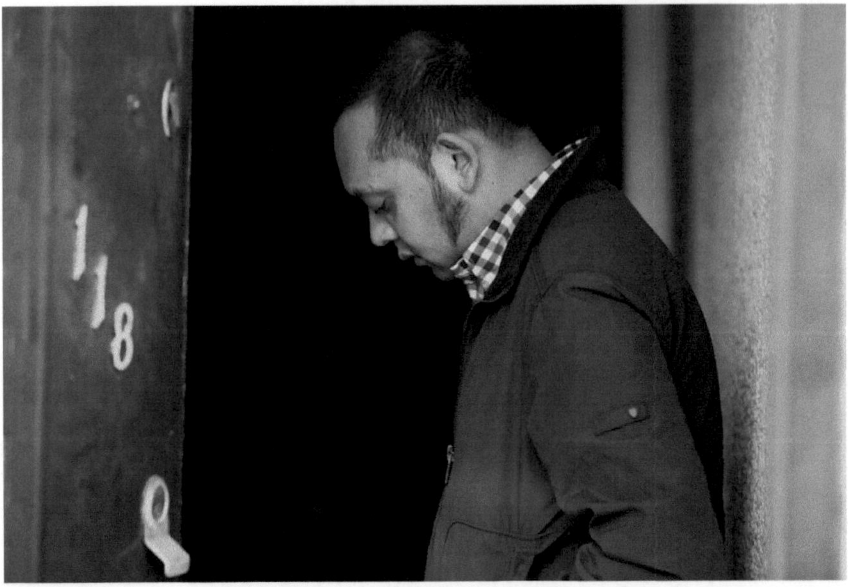

Figure 8.4 Gillian Wearing *Self Made* (2010) colour film with sound, 84 minutes. © Gillian Wearing, courtesy Maureen Paley, London.

real, the appearance of an authentic self beyond the impersonations of social appearances? The camera moves in closer, the film playing to the viewer's curiosity. Rumbelow, as if he is a mediumistic channel for the cathartic purgation of Ash's emotions, lays his hands solemnly on his shoulders. Such a reading of the scene would align more with a straightforwardly therapeutic idea of release through art, whereas I want to claim that something more dynamic might be happening in which the conflictual is being treated, but not eradicated, by re-enacting conflict. Although the political and social context of Augusto Boal's *Theatre of the Oppressed* is far removed from this scenario,[27] his view on the meanings of catharsis in theatre is useful to considering the film scene I have just described as part of a process of self-actualization that is not simply curative. This tallies with a Boalian aesthetic the goal of which is 'to "create chaos" and establish a "healthy disorder" […] disaligning […] therapeutic values from notions of unification, conformity, adaptation, harmony, cohesion' (Schutzman, 1994: 148).

For Boal, the cathartic process, as inherited from Aristotelian theatre, has to do with a purgation of fear and pity.[28] In this model, catharsis has to do with the correction and purification of nature. The actor arouses terror and pity in the audience in order to cure them of those emotions, leading Boal to conclude that Aristotelian theatre is a 'powerful system of intimidation', its basic task being 'the purgation of all antisocial elements' (2008: 40). Interestingly, this purgation is homeopathically induced, Boal citing Milton that 'in physick medicine, things of melancholick hue and quality are used against melancholy, sour against sour, salt to remove salt humours' (2008: 27). For Boal, and in my pharmacological argument, cathartic purgation is problematic as it results in a reinstatement of the status quo, both pacifying the audience and making them feel vindicated through their empathetic identification with the protagonist. However, might a homeopathic purgation offer something else? Not the 'awakening of critical consciousness' (Boal, 2008: 98) that Brecht put forward as a corrective to Aristotelian catharsis, and which Boal finds limiting, as do I, in that contemporary media implicitly perform critique to appeal to and mirror contemporary audiences' savvy.[29] But rather an aesthetic space in which toxicity, in being homeopathically treated by exacerbation, results in a purgation that creates a 'healthy disorder' that is nonetheless transformative?[30]

While Boal's Latin American context was bound up with a radical leftist pedagogy in which acting as a 'poetics of the oppressed' (2008: 98) entailed the transformation of spectators into protagonists trained for real action, i.e. social revolution, his idea of training for action has broader implications. For Boal, as Daniel Feldhendler adumbrates, theatre 'emerges in the moment in which the human being recognizes that s/he can see himself or herself [...]; s/he recognizes who s/he is and is not; s/he imagines who s/he could become' (1994: 93–4). Training for action can also be applied to theatre as an aesthetic space in which inner psychic realities are explored by means of the dissociative gap between the subject as both actor and spectator of their own performance. Boal uses the term 'spect-actor' to refer to theatre as the art of looking at ourselves in which we are at one and the same time actor and spectator. It could be said that within *Self Made* participants are transformed into Boalian 'spect-actors', being the creative protagonists of their own dramatic scenarios, in which they are both acting and observing themselves acting rather than simply purging negative emotions.[31] This redirects *Self Made* from simply being considered a coercive film that manipulates its 'working-class' participants and its mainly art audience. Just as Boal's spect-actors would enact scenarios from life to try and find solutions to everyday problems, *Self Made*'s participants ultimately discover their own resources to deal with emotional issues through their fictional re-enactments. While participants in a film such as *Self Made*, unlike Boalian theatre, are separate from their audience, nonetheless the projection of their performances show that people have innate knowledge of how to become spect-actors if given the opportunity. Rather than seeing this as a capitulation to the neoliberal injunction to become better selves, I read *Self Made*'s participants' creative inventions as transformative experiences of selfhood in which subjects become, to paraphrase an infamous Lacanian proverb, that which they shall have been in the process of becoming all along.[32] For me, this is exemplified by Ash's 'end film'.

Before training for this film, Ash speaks direct-to-camera about his choice to play a role where he kicks a pregnant woman in the street and kills her baby. He says that this scenario is the worst he could imagine, as if implying that such an enactment might be a homeopathic purging of the abuse he suffered as a child, an issue which he confessed in a previous workshop. The editing in *Self Made* is extremely elliptical, so the only build-up the viewer has to Ash's choice of scenario is some footage of a training session in which Ash repeatedly kicks a pig carcass, Rumbelow encouraging him to situate his action in relation to past bodies he would have liked to hit. The imagined other as target of violence transforms the carcass into an object that is *used* to act out the emotion in the present. Ash breaks down, the initial feeling of enjoying his power over the carcass converting to feeling bad about the violent emotions he has imbibed from witnessing domestic abuse and being beaten by his stepfather as a child. At first, akin to the previous scene, it might appear that Ash's breakdown is a cathartic release of emotion rather than a step in the process of becoming able to play with emotional trauma. As the camera closes in on Ash's breakdown, the vulnerability of the documentary subject in their willing subjection to the camera's interrogation is made palpably discomforting, which is why I think Wearing intermittently inserts what I consider to be clichéd moments of reflexivity in the film, as if doing so rescues its inherent toxicity. But paradoxically, what Ash's 'end film' exposes is not the pseudo-criticality of the making of a documentary or the cathartic outpouring that would enable a viewer to empathize and pity, but rather how the performative testing out of emotions generates the self-scrutiny to enable personal transformation. In other words, the capacity to make emotions into objects to be used in the Winnicottian sense, i.e. creatively destroyed, so that the subject can separate from previous inhibiting identifications. This does not mean they are cured, but that they can more easily tolerate inner conflict so that it becomes productive rather than inhibiting. This idea also seems close to Boal's notion of training for real action whereby catharsis is replaced by the creation of what he calls 'a sort of uneasy sense of incompleteness' (Boal, 2008: 119). The latter is what must be tolerated in the human being's journey from what Winnicott calls 'identicality' to 'separation' that I referred to in Chapter 6. It is also useful to recall the characteristics of Winnicott's transitional object here: the object is irrational from the perspective of the adult and it survives all kinds of cruelty, thereby enabling boundaries to be redrawn that are invisible to the observing adult. The analogy I'm making vis-à-vis Ash's worst-case scenario is that it functions like a transitional space in relation to which the spectator outside the film is a bit like the observing adult who, not liking what they see, might judge the action on moral grounds rather than viewing it as part of a psychic act of creative destruction that is partly inaccessible to the observer.

Something, however, is made accessible to the viewer. In performing his 'end film', Ash was having difficulty channelling the remorse he felt he should feel after hitting a pregnant woman, the sonic impact of which shocks the viewer's senses much as the idea itself is abhorrent, though it is the case that these desires exist and are acted on in society. By repeating them in a staged context, Ash is unwittingly engaging in a form of critique in which art mimics 'reality' both to show its injurious nature and to potentially liberate the self from unreflective acting-out. This is Method's homeopathic potential, but the performance, I would say, goes further than merely treating like with like. Rounding the corner after his violent action, Ash attempts to cry but eventually calls a halt to the filming, upset that he cannot feel the remorse appropriate to the heinous nature of the act. The crew and cameras are shown on-screen and Rumbelow is called on set to help Ash reconnect with the emotional places they explored in the workshops. Reiterating this role-play enables Ash to act out the requisite emotion. For me, this display that the technique is a construction does not destroy its 'truth-effect' in producing remorse. The 'truth-effect', which bypasses the ideology of emotion that would naturalize it as an authentic outpouring of a volitional subject, happens in two worlds at the same time, the fictive world of the film and the psychic world of Ash's processing of the emotion. Taking a Deleuzian approach to this film, David Deamer reaches a similar conclusion saying that in relation to the participants and their characters '[w]e have not reached some inner truth. They have gone out of themselves, made new connections, *false truths*' (2012: 44, my emphasis). This kind of Deleuzian-inspired depersonalization of emotion transverses one's interpellation as a raced, classed and/or gendered subject, enhancing one's capacity to explore the creative potential of being.

Ash had introduced himself as an immigrant to Newcastle in the 1980s who suffered racial as well as domestic abuse. In a cogent reading of *Self Made*, Jenny Chamarette reads his performance as stemming from 'the difference of his experiences, as working class, as a self-defined immigrant, as an abused child', though she is quick to acknowledge that his performance also enables spectators to 'reflect on affect as a mode of exploring the creative power of difference' (2015: 139). To my mind, Chamarette is alluding to two kinds of difference here: one being social difference, the other being difference as a creative act in which one's social interpellation is exceeded. This would be akin to Deamer's notion that the participants make 'new connections'. It is here that one becomes open to the aesthetic promise of change without denying the toxicity it brings in its train. The pharmacological nature of this aesthetic training can be further highlighted by contrasting Ash's post 'end film' reflections to those of another of the participants, Lian, with which I shall conclude this chapter.

Lian, who coincidently looks a lot like Wearing, had enacted a theatrical scene from Shakespeare's *King Lear* in which his daughter, Cordelia, challenges and confronts her father, the scene being analogous to abandonment issues Lian had with her father. In a Boalian sense, it could be said that she is using theatrical emotions to cure analogous problems in her life. In Lian's post 'end film' reflection, she is shown in mid-shot standing at the window inside her flat, wistfully looking out, while her voice-over tells us that things are now better between herself and her father. She is then shown speaking direct-to-camera affirming that now 'I know he loves me' and 'He texts us everyday'. Lian's sense of self-recovery fits more with the management of emotions in which negativity is banished and the self is shored up by positive feeling. The off-screen Lian may indeed feel positive about her relation to her father after her performance, but for the viewer, her self-assurance does not evidence a gap between the self she presents as 'cured' and the self as a work of incompleteness. Ash's slippage between the real and the feigned in his use of Method techniques is more suggestive of the possibility to engage in acts of self-scrutiny that might have a less predictable outcome. Method enables Ash to distribute his fictive, real and imagined selves in scenarios in which other 'actors', e.g. Ash's mother and stepfather, do not necessarily remain locked in the same places as victims and/or perpetrators, but are assembled in psychic constellations that play with negative disabling emotions, transforming them without getting rid of them. Method and REBT are technical tools that can be used to create performances of identity whose outcomes are potentially curative without denying the toxicity of damaging experiences. Rather than, as Horning puts it, bewailing the 'loss of personal integrity and dignity entailed by impersonations of social existence' (2013), these impersonations could be said to act as an aesthetic treatment of the psychological disorders that stem from the privations of neoliberal governance without these acts simply being an acquisition of social capital or self-aggrandizement. Such enactments of 'fictional truths' might enable more liveable lives off the radar of 'achievement society'.

9

The transitional pleasures of emotional labour in Lucy Beech's and Rehana Zaman's videos

The view that cognitive capitalism is characterized by a modality that 'amplifies, accelerates and captures our biological, emotional and intellectual force in order to convert them to profit' (Zepke in Braidotti and Pisters, 2012: 218) can be given yet another slant if thought specifically in relation to gendered and racialized subjects. The artists' moving image works I focus on in this chapter by Lucy Beech and Rehana Zaman cast other perspectives on how resistance might operate by mimicking neoliberal discourses of self-improvement and aspiration. The therapeutic aesthetics of Beech's and Zaman's films imagine life-enhancing potential within the exploitative conditions of cognitive or semiocapitalism. In this they can be aligned with Berardi's notion that 'aesthetics seems to be at the same time a diagnostic of the psychospheric pollution and a therapy for the relation between organism and its world' (2009: 130). The particular relation between organism and world that I shall examine in their films is the feminized condition of immaterial labour whereby, for those subjects who are bound to the reproductive care that capitalism depends on for production, Berardi's Autonomist call for the withdrawal of labour is not an option. In both Beech's and Zaman's films, resistance has to be thought from within the sphere of production and in relation to cognitive and affective subjugation. Before embarking on my analysis of the artists' films, I want to briefly account for why that is.

Regardless of the fact that women have entered the realm of productive labour in their hoards, there is still a separation between the immaterial labour that is necessary for the maintenance of the species and the immaterial labour from which surplus value can be extracted and exchanged on the market place. The necessity of immaterial labour in the home for example is still largely invisible to capital. It is assumed that either a working woman pays for this work to be done or she combines it with paid labour. For some feminists, the invisibility of reproductive labour paradoxically offers some respite from the battleground of productive labour. For example, as well as mundane repetition, child-rearing also affords joys that are incommensurable with the quantification of value and time that the productive sphere imposes on bodies. Paradoxically too, the reification in the private sphere of joy in being with children is somewhat echoed in Berardi's romantic positing of the affective and linguistic bond between mother and child as a resistance to the logic of recombinant flux that characterizes cognitive or semiocapitalism in that, for him, it preserves poetic forms of conjunction rather than the disruption of digital connection (2017). As I discussed in Chapter 5, it is this linguistic form of conjunction that he sees as being destroyed in semiocapitalism now that machines, rather than mothers, entrain infants, sentiments that chime somewhat with Stiegler's view of the colonization of the maternal-environment of transitional space. However, as Silvia Federici says: 'reproductive labour has always been a problem for autonomist theories of labour' (2006). As she sees it, the concept of affective labour promulgated by Berardi, Virno and Negri, rather than being a terrain of struggle and a site of solidarity between the immaterial labour performed by cognitive capitalism's neuro-workers and the unpaid, or poorly paid, domestic labourers capitalism depends on, instead 'brings reproductive work back into the world of mystification' (2006). Her point is that the theory of precarious and immaterial labour only speaks to the situation and interest of workers working at the highest level of capitalistic technology. While I agree with Federici's premise, her call for the formation of collective movements whose objective would be to share responsibility for the maintenance and care of all spheres of labour is beyond the scope of my book. Rather, in bringing moving image works by female artists addressing affective labour into a conjunction with the therapeutic as both curative and toxic, I shall explore how subjectification might also afford transitional moments of liberation. Feminist philosopher Rosi Braidotti's strategy of affirmation is conducive to this pharmacological modality of aesthetics. Braidotti says that:

> political agency need not be critical in the negative sense of oppositional and thus may not be aimed solely or primarily at the production of counter-

> subjectivities. Subjectivity is rather a process ontology of auto-poiesis or self-styling, which involves complex and continuous negotiations with dominant norms and values. (in Dolphijn and van der Tuin, 2012)

Opportunities for 'self-styling' through affective labour have increased in neoliberal cognitive capitalism. Self-improvement through wellness, fitness and therapy regimes, while serving capital, also afford opportunities for women, albeit of a certain class, to assemble and perform group work in which they might acquire a provisional autonomy that is not simply subservient to capital or a means of professional development. Aspects of this conflictual complicity can be seen in Beech's work, which predominantly features white middle- to lower-middle-class women, but it can also be thought more globally, as occurs in Zaman's film. In bringing these two artists' work together, my goal is to intimate something along the lines of Donna Haraway's coalitions between women of different class, race and gender for the sake of creating an imaginary of situated 'partial perspectives' (1988: 584). Haraway's ethos of 'partial perspectives' is a counterpoint to absolutist perspectives and remedies as well as to 'bulldozer' concepts. For example, as Zechner and Rübner Hansen point out in their review of Stiegler's *For a New Critique of Political Economy* (2012): 'The absence of a feminist and postcolonial viewpoint – or even recognition thereof – does make itself felt in Stiegler's work, and with this, questions of care and sustainability become somewhat shallow' (2012). For them, and I agree, Stiegler's notion of care 'is blind to how any mode of care is internally and antagonistically split according to class, gender and race' (2012). They raise the point that Stiegler's

> 'economy of contribution' sits rather awkwardly historically with women, who whether as mothers, wives, witches or prostitutes have developed and passed on an incredible wealth of knowledges and practices of care and communisation, despite having no access to mainstream institutions, public spaces or high technologies. It also sits strangely with cultures that haven't yet gone through quite as many cycles of accumulation to arrive at the techno-individual of Stiegler's narrative. (2012)

Remaining with the remit of my book to explore the pharmacological aesthetics of moving image artworks in relation to transitional spaces, in what follows, I examine how Beech's and Zaman's feminist-inspired narratives of toxicity and cure straddle conflictual spaces of female solidarity and care in the nexus of global and cognitive capitalism in a UK context.

> I am my own enterprise, if Fordism integrated consumption into the cycle of capitalism, post-Fordism integrates reproduction and communication … subjectivity is the raw material for immaterial labour.[1]

Post-Fordism can be aligned with the kind of labour which (re)produces 'immaterial goods such as a service, a cultural product, knowledge or communication' (Hardt and Negri, 2001: 290). However, material labour does not disappear. It continues both in the Global North's outsourcing of assembly-line Fordism to so-called less developed countries and in the employment of cheap migrant labour. However, the fact that all forms of labour in cognitive capitalism are increasingly dependent on the immaterial attributes of communication and emotion has expanded the areas of life available for the extraction of capital value. As opposed to Marxist analyses of Fordist industrial labour where maintenance of the sphere of reproduction was relegated to an unsalaried, largely female, invisible workforce, in a post-Fordist, cognitive capitalist economy, while maintenance of the reproductive sphere of the home is still an issue, its affective ecology of care and labour has transmuted into a new source of capital to be extracted from all workers from call centre operatives to freelance creatives. While Federici, as I have said, is critical of theorists of immaterial labour for not recognizing the power relations at work in the 'feminist analysis of the function of the sexual division of labor' (2006),[2] other theorists argue that these new conditions of exploitation also harness new political subjectivities which might be capable of releasing 'a social potential for transformation, largely attributable to [their] affective dimensions and the opportunities for human contact and interaction' (Gill and Pratt, 2008: 8). Within the exploitative conditions they image, both Beech's and Zaman's films envision the potentiality of female group solidarity as an uncommodified pleasure and value that might provide momentary glimpses of such transformation. In this, their therapeutic aesthetics moves beyond being diagnostic, but neither is it purely remedial, my argument being that while moving image artwork can proffer models of solidarity, it does not solve problems.

Beech's series of films since 2013 idiosyncratically reflect on economies of female aspiration in cognitive capitalism. In videos such as *Cannibals* (2013), *Me and Mine* (2015) and *Pharmakon* (2016) as well as two five-minute videos from 2013, *Well Being* and *Buried Alive*,[3] Beech presents conflictual sites of female subjectivity in which the desire for transformation is frequently equivalent, not to political democracy and equality, but to entrepreneurial business models and the use of reskilling as a resource to achieve financial as well as personal success. In her three films from 2013 which I shall mainly refer to, ridding oneself of negative emotions and addictions is held out as a promise of a life that is more financially and personally rewarding. At the same time, engaging in some form of therapeutic life coaching to achieve this better life also seems to exacerbate the neurotic compulsions that drive the women to seek transformation in the first place. In a general sense, one might say that the characters in the films exemplify the poisonous adaptive model of marketization that for Stiegler short-circuits the transmission of knowledge across generations. But, given that Stiegler's analysis does not consider feminist perspectives, his monolithic view of adaptation fails to see that for subjects who are already considered somewhat poisonous in relation to the dominant patriarchal orders of power, i.e. women, adaptation might involve its own transitional pleasures of transmission.

Interestingly, although the film is in no way an application of Stiegler's ideas, Beech refers in passing to Stiegler's *What Makes Life Worth Living* in her film notes for *Pharmakon*, the bulk of her research for that film being into the phenomenon of Delusional Infestation and Morgellons disease, a skin condition which the protagonist of her film suffers from. Although Morgellons is sometimes manifest on the surface of the skin as rashes, sufferers' sensations of crawling, biting and stinging mostly occur below the surface of the skin invisible to the eye. In this, as a metaphor at least, it seems an apt symptom to join the plethora of other pathological symptoms that are said by Stiegler, Han and Berardi to be exacerbated in cognitive capitalism, i.e. ADHD, anxiety, depression, panic, etc. The other aspect of Morgellons that metaphorically epitomizes the connectivity of the digital age is that its symptoms, which include fatigue, are highly contagious via online forums for sharing illness in the network economy. Diagnosed by the medical profession as delusional psychosis, treatment is by drugs, but dissatisfied and marginalized by mainstream medicine, sufferers form online communities to self-diagnose, prescribe and purchase alternative therapeutic treatments.[4] Beech's film notes are telling, documenting that:

> clinician's working within the field of psychiatry consider connectivity in this context as destructive and generative in equal measure. Antagonistic toward these online groups, many acknowledge that the community is a virtual space of collective vindication sustaining and even giving rise to the itch. The itch in this sense is adopted within the framework of the film as a means of exploring contagion as a social process.[5]

It is as if the internet acts like a virtual clinic in which these female sufferers perform their symptoms for one another rather than for a room full of male doctors as in Jean-Martin Charcot's infamous sessions at Salpêtrière hospital in the nineteenth century in which so-called hysterics performed their uncanny symptoms as spectacle. Hysteria came to signify a mode of contagious female behaviours whose force could not be tamed by patriarchal control, yet, at the same time such control engendered the hysterical body's revolt. Although I am speculating here, it is not a great leap of the imagination to see Morgellons as a symptom, at least in a metaphorical sense, of female subjection to the conditions and dictates of neoliberal capitalism to self-improve and be successful in a competitive environment. Sufferers turn to the theatre of the internet for emotional and pharmaceutical support, both of which provide solace but also exacerbate the level of addiction to the disease as the defining marker of sufferers' identities, the soft marketing of profitable alternative remedies preying on their vulnerability.

Pharmakon's silent central protagonist, FB, is a female bouncer who believes she is suffering from the disease. Modelled on Renée Jeanne Falconetti, the star of Carl Theodor Dreyer's *The Passion of Joan of Arc* (1928), her silent stoicism conveys scepticism, despair and hope, as she engages in various entrainment behaviours, including a workshop on energy contact training, a martial arts method of bringing someone to a stop without touching them. In her quest to alleviate her invisible symptoms, she logs into a meditation video distributed by The Healing Grapevine, an alternative healing centre run by entrepreneur Christa. Initially, FB acts as a sceptical foil to the display of positive energy exuded by Christa, especially in the promotional video she makes to market the centre. In her role as sceptical observer, which I see as a kind of stand-in for the viewer, FB remains on the outskirts of the clinic's therapy group 'me-time' session. But, perhaps due to an escalation of her symptoms, by the end of the film she joins the assembly of fellow sufferers and imbibes the company's curative cleansing water that promises to heal the women's symptoms from the inside out. This promise and the solidarity of the all-female group are seductive protections against the harshness of potential aggression in FB's life, both in her job as a bouncer and in relation to the uncontrollable irritation under her skin. The proliferation of screens within screens in the film, for example, Christa's promotional video is projected on a screen at the assembly as well as on FB's phone, encourages a reading of how pharmacological adaptation spreads toxicity. *Pharmakon* neither condemns the exploitative nature of this business nor celebrates the fact that, unlike nineteenth-century hysterics, women in the twenty-first century can self-organize, albeit under the auspices of the market.[6] There seems to be no escape from the cyclical ritual of cleansing and toxicity and its connection to profit. In this the film could be said to offer a less collective spirit than Beech's films from 2013, her work seeming to move from the conflictual group solidarities of the latter to the representation of more solitary heroines isolated amongst groups of women.

As opposed to this, *Well Being* and *Buried Alive* which are often shown together, as well as the longer short film *Cannibals*, gesture more towards a sense of solidarity and the pleasure of group work for the aspirational women that congregate within them. The group in *Cannibals* consists of white, lower-middle to middle-class women who belong to a do-it-yourself pyramid investment scheme, loosely based on the real-life online pyramid community 'Women Empowering Women' (WEW), which was one of many schemes of this ilk popular in the 1990s. The pyramids comprised groups of eight women who would each be recruited to invest £3000 in the scheme. Once the group was complete, the leader would then gain £24,000 and move on to allow the recruits below her in the pyramid to complete their own group, the goal being that each investor would recoup and make a huge profit from their initial investment. The UK government tried to put a ban on these groups in 2001 as, of course, while a few women succeeded, many, unable to recruit their own groups, simply lost their investment. Beech's video features six women congregating in the group leader's garden-flat for a feast to which they bring the dishes that represent their place in the pyramid; for example, newcomers bring starters, the leader, the dessert. During the course of the meeting, the women perform a series of ritualistic, ostensibly therapeutic, behaviours in the hope of exorcizing inhibiting memories and rising higher in the triangle. As Beech intends, and this was certainly my experience of viewing the video, *Cannibals* can be read as an allegory of female immaterial labour under global capitalism in which women are encouraged to be their own entrepreneurs, to be aspirational and self-improving as well as responsible for their own well-being. Whereas the real-life context of the pyramid community WEW was explicitly bound up in the acquisition of money, *Cannibals* adapts its ethos of being an all-female support group and gears it towards effecting psychological rather than purely financial transformation. No money is glimpsed in the film. Instead, the collapsing of the psychological into the financial is played out in the rituals undergone by the six women in the marquee in group leader Helen's garden. Sitting in a group circle, the women engage in a psychodramatic ritual to reinforce positive thought in the present.

Helen refers to this ritual as 'emotional circuit training', 'a marinating process', which softens and breaks down connective tissue, loosening the body to make it ready to receive the benefits of the pyramid. The women place electrodes on their bodies, Helen makes a salt gargle and another woman lights

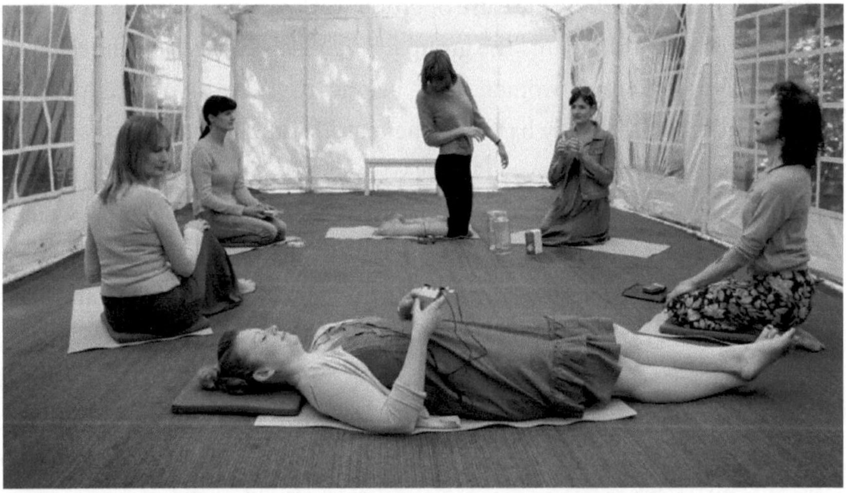

Figure 9.1 Lucy Beech, *Cannibals*, 2013. Video still. Courtesy of the artist.

up a cigarette while Dorothy, the sceptical counterfoil to Helen's enthusiasm, is given the speakers mat. She recounts a fear of ascending the upper floors of a building. She wants the money to buy a bungalow, but also fears climbing up in case of a crash. The allusion to a crash is suggestive of either a financial or an emotional risk, her monologue here pointing to how in the context of neoliberal capitalism, the two go hand in hand. As Catherine Rottenberg, citing Wendy Brown, says: '[o]ne of the hallmarks of our neoliberal age is precisely the casting of every human endeavor and activity in entrepreneurial terms' (2014: 421). As the economic and the emotional coalesce in Dorothy's monologue, the group members engage in a collective paroxysm of hysterical trembling as if incorporating and expulsing Dorothy's fears from the inside. Helen gargles the saltwater, the other woman exhales cigarette smoke, salting and smoking both actions associated with curing flesh, curing in this context being a pun on healing. Dorothy's voice-over, the only one in the film, begins when she swops places to take up the role of cigarette smoker, a ritual usually considered damaging but here the smoke is considered transformative, the poisonous toxins effecting a curative purging from deep within the body. As Dorothy ruminates on this inverse healing, the next woman up on the speaker's mat confesses her addiction to online poker. The psychodramatic role-playing in which the group are encouraged to see themselves as characters to gain a perspective on their problems and desires,[7] culminates in a feast loosely inspired by Mikhail Bakhtin's carnivalesque, a concept of festival in which hierarchies are overturned. Identifying with the foodstuffs that represent their place in the pyramid – they are by turns garlic bread, prawn dumplings and a blini – the women metaphorically consume themselves, as if the process of ingesting this food will free them from the internal constraints that prevent their success. Beech refers to this as an allegory of capitalism, stating that the work is 'a microcosm of a capitalist system, mirroring an image of unsustainable growth' (in Nunes, 2015). The women's desire to self-improve and succeed incorporates them more thoroughly in an endless cycle of self-exploitation that can only escalate until it implodes. In the real-life phenomenon, this would occur with some of the women on the bottom losing all their money, while the leader creams off the rewards. In *Cannibals*, the implosion occurs from within the body. As Dorothy observes with insight, 'we are consuming ourselves.' Her face merges into her plate of blinis, while her internal monologue rapidly recites a speech which is a cut-up of statements from a WEW website and quotes from Bahktin's *Rabelais and his World*.[8] Honing in on the feast, the camera lingers on the food going into the women's mouths, its being chewed and swallowed in a grotesque inverse of the 'food porn' of contemporary supermarket advertising. Reversing the seductive luxuriating of close-ups of overpriced convenience food in such advertising, the self-devouring occurring in the feast exemplifies the entropy at work in consumption and drags this profit-motivated aspirational labour into the realm of the reproductive, i.e. that which needs to be done all over again to maintain life. Rather than simply a microcosm of the capitalist system at large, the women's actions can be specifically related to the condition of the feminist neoliberal subject under contemporary cognitive capitalism in which many of the demands of previous generations of feminists for equality and autonomy in economic and social life are sold back to a current generation as personal, rather than social, imperatives and forms of governance. As Rottenberg diagnoses, the neoliberal feminist subject 'accepts full responsibility for her own well-being and self-care' (2014: 420), thereby disavowing the social, cultural and economic forces that produce inequality.

Beech has said that '[t]he therapeutic potential of the group's haptic communication is negated by the meetings internal hierarchies that mirror a capitalist model' (in Nunes, 2015). However, while the belief that you alone are responsible for your own well-being wins out in the end – and it is noteworthy that in the final sequence Helen puts her *intact* pavlova back in the freezer – an alternative energy and collective solidarity are suggested between the women through their transpersonal capacities to feel one another's emotions. In this way, *Cannibals* proposes a relational psychological body, which exceeds the calculating, self-regulating, hierarchical structure of the capitalist triangle and squanders its surplus in a foolish, perhaps joyous, act of collective self-consumption. Herein lies the film's pharmacological therapeutic aesthetics, the uselessness of foolish squandering remedying the excess of positivity necessary to be a successful entrepreneur.

Although only approximately five minutes in duration both *Well Being* and *Buried Alive* perform a pharmacological implosion of positivity. Both films show group learning situations in which bodily techniques are deployed as a means of freeing emotional blockage. In *Well Being*, a number of white middle-aged, lower-middle to middle-class women attend a workshop on how to deal with negative emotions like shame through performative body work. The workshop leader gives forth on how these techniques will be useful to participants in their future roles as group leaders, the goal being to transform negative emotions into an object that can be picked up, felt, tasted, smelled and thereby released. While some of the women engage in the body work demonstrations on offer in the suburban front room – these include movements akin to reiki and shiatsu as well as a kind of therapeutic shaking, all overseen by the leader/therapist – one woman constantly roams around the room taking photos of the demos on her phone. Again, she appears to be the sceptical foil to the leader's upbeat rhetoric about reclaiming one's emotional body. Beech's camerawork reinforces her implied critique of the workshop. As this woman finally lies on the floor to participate, the film takes her lopsided point-of-view of the room, as if formally questioning the leadership model.

It is with some surprise that the sceptical woman reappears as the workshop leader in *Buried Alive*. The film opens on a mid-shot of four women digging a hole on a beach. It cuts to an interior in which the leader is explaining that the workshop will explore strategies for eradicating guilt. Back on the beach, one of the women lies down into the hole while the others cover her over. This therapeutic action is reminiscent of Lygia Clark's *Baba Antropofagica* (Anthropophagic Slobber) (1973),[9] in which a group of people were instructed to put a spool of coloured thread in their mouths, then cover the entire body of the group member who lies blindfolded at the centre with the moistened strands. Violently tearing away the saliva-moistened cocoon to release the body, Clark's psychotherapeutic art event proposed a collective healing whereby all members of the group can be renewed through the metaphoric cannibalization of the body at the centre of the activity. In releasing them from the cocoon, the group expels their inner toxicity. But in Beech's rendition of group burial, the goal is positive affirmation, not abject confrontation with the other. The woman's head protrudes like Millais' *Ophelia* (1851–1852), but there is no tragic dimension to this 'death'. It is enacted in a matter-of-fact manner and with little further ado, the other women dig her out again to the accompaniment of encouraging comments like 'well done'. A supportive group clap welcomes her as she returns from a cleansing dip in the ocean.

According to psychologist Silvan Tomkins, guilt and shame are the main emotions that destroy and/or hold us back from making connections (Sedgwick 2003). By performing techniques in which the body symbolically buries those emotions, the implication is that connections to the world can be remade. In *Buried Alive*, these emotional connections are propped on a business model in which women can go on to lead their own well-being workshops. However, there is also a kind of empathetic solidarity between the women that is not purely economic and stems from the pleasure of group activity and its potential to redistribute emotional conflicts so that they become less identified with individuals.

As I have previously described, the notion of well-being in contemporary society has become a value subscribed to and heralded by governments at the same time that funding public resources that might provide such flourishing are cut. The responsibility for achieving well-being and the idea that well-being is something to be achieved rather than nurtured are put squarely in the hands of the individual. It is seen as a commodity in an economy in which negative emotions such as depression and anxiety are a drain. The entry of well-being into the market not only makes it the preserve of classes of people with the financial resources to acquire it, but also exacerbates the tendency for people without those resources to channel their grievances and problems into other parts of the service industries such as call centres. The affective labour, mainly female, call centre workers are called upon to provide increases their stress levels that in turn necessitate self-medication and/or self-care to enable one to continue to provide the service that one depends on for a living regardless of its transformation into a form of therapeutic reproductive labour that exceeds one's pay grade. Corporate in-house therapies such as counselling and away days act as buffers to manage stress-related symptoms, the provision of such remedies adding to the image of the corporation as a caring entity and thereby preventing scrutiny of how its capitalization of emotional labour might generate the very illnesses its employees are exhorted to self-manage.

This context forms the backdrop to the scenario enacted in Zaman's short film *5* (2014), in which five women, who work in a call centre, are on an away day in the suburban countryside, getting out of the office being seen as a natural remedy for stress and thereby a means of enhancing productivity. While in Beech's films, group work tends towards members performing activities that stand-in for psychological symptoms, in 5, group work is dominated by one of the women's on-screen narrative voice, as she recounts stories about the ubiquity of receiving sex calls on what is a suicide helpline. The other women either interject the odd question or contribute one-liners to complete her story as if they were all different parts of her psyche rather than individuals in their own right. Shots of the women floating down the river, Ophelia-like, are intercut with the collective monologue, their meaning becoming clearer in the final part of the film where the women white-out one another's faces as if in preparation for a theatrical performance or a ritualistic cleansing. Akin to Beech's films, the whole scenario and its absurd denouement are enacted in a matter-of-fact, non-dramatic manner. As the women float downstream, an act which could be seen as a performative death akin to the burial scene in *Buried Alive*, a question arises as to whether these acts of renewal are the means by which the effects of (self) exploitation can be mitigated or whether their relation to labour is more ambiguous, suggesting, as they do, a form of oneiric withdrawal from productivity that recalls Berardi's aforementioned proposal as well as my introductory encounter with Rist's *Worry Will Vanish Horizon*.

Withdrawal from the sphere of work is not an option in Zaman's *Some Women, Other Women and All the Bittermen* (2014). While speaking to the ramifications of women's immaterial labour in global capitalism, the film does not explicitly mimic a therapeutic scenario; however, it does suggest the necessity of thinking self-cultivation beyond the preserve of the cognitariat or expanding middle classes. *Some Women, Other Women and All the Bittermen* was initially exhibited as a gallery installation on six monitors that spatially replicated the episodic format of a soap drama, though it can be viewed as a single-screen work of forty-nine minutes' duration which is how I encountered it.[10] Zaman based her invented soap on the 1990s international takeover of Tetley brewery and each of the six episodes, as screened on the monitors, also included documentary footage of workshops she participated in with the self-organized group *Justice for Domestic Workers* (J4DW) (Leeds). The group, who since 2018 are called 'The Voice of Domestic Workers', is a self-help, grassroots organization made up of multi-national, migrant domestic workers in the UK.[11] While it may seem trite to juxtapose the real conditions of oppression that the, largely Asian, domestic workers operate under with the fictional women in Beech's film who have the leisure to self-exploit, it is my contention that the conditions of immaterial labour in which the cognitive and emotional capacities of subjectivity are mined as 'raw material' have multifarious effects which need to be thought in conjunction with one another. In part, Zaman's juxtapositioning of the soap opera with the footage of J4DW meetings underscores this, her video making an intervention in the lack of literature addressing 'the specific case of bodies marked by gender and race' (Charlesworth, 2015: 89) in discourses on immaterial labour in the art world and in Autonomist philosophy.

There is an obvious level on which the plight of foreign domestic workers in the UK is interlinked with the immaterial labour of an aspirational middle-class female workforce. As Charlesworth, citing art historian Angela Dimitrakaki, says: 'women's increased presence in the paid workforce has not been facilitated by a redistribution of task or through state support in the sphere of social reproduction, but rather the site of exploitation has shifted to (largely) female migrant workers' (91). Rather than further exploring the social inequality that underpins this, it is my contention that what Lütticken calls the 'neoliberal theatre' of post-Fordist production – in which 'it became imperative to present oneself not so much as an interchangeable supplier of labour-power [...] but to perform oneself as a unique commodity-person' (2005: 17) – is not exclusive to a white lower-middle to middle-class. In this sense, Haraway's *Simians, Cyborgs and Women: The Reinvention of Nature*, first published in 1991, is newly resonant in its articulation of how all workers under global capitalism are subject to vexed social relations between women and machines, labour and care. Haraway's prescient situating of women of colour, white socialist feminism and technological capitalism on a continuum acts as a corrective to the current largely ungendered discourses of immaterial labour. Describing what I would call the pharmacological nature of women's opportunities for integration and exploitation in the new global conditions of machine labour, she says:

> The home, workplace, market, public arena, the body itself – all can be dispersed and interfaced in nearly infinite, polymorphous ways, with large consequences for women and others – consequences that themselves are very different for different people and which make potent positional interrelational movements *difficult to imagine* and *essential for survival.* (1991: 163, my emphasis)

To begin the difficult task of imagining the possibility of such alliances, it is necessary to think across the multiple material effects of this economy without, of course, blurring the distinctions between them.

By juxtaposing a soap drama about the Tetley takeover with the documentary present of the domestic workers, Zaman's video begins to do this. The soap features a British male working-class soon to be disposed of in a corporate takeover and focuses on the main female protagonist, Sue, an ambitious secretary, who repeatedly comes up against sexism. The brewery manager Colin refuses to promote her to management until he realizes he has to get rid of 'dead weight' in preparation for the takeover. Sue's supposedly feminine reproductive attributes of being caring and empathetic are then seen as a valued asset. Inserting the documentary footage into the soap episodes, the film contrasts the erosion of white, male, industrial labour in a globalized market with a labour force comprising women of colour, two groups who are now no longer geographically separated as they were in the 1990s when Haraway was writing about the production of a 'new world-wide working class, as well as new sexualities and ethnicities' (1991: 166).

In the 1990s too, there was a shift in Western feminist discourse from an emphasis on activism to one on cultural critique in which the pleasures of soap opera audiences, largely female homemakers, were revalued as worthy of academic attention.[12] As opposed to dismissing soap operas as a form of working-class entertainment that contrasts to the supposedly superior viewing of high art, feminist media scholar Charlotte Brunsdon, also a key reference for Zaman, reread the pleasures of soap opera in terms of a latent critique of patriarchy. Aside from their portrayal of strong female characters, soaps, in constituting largely female audiences as expert interpreters of their moral universes, could be seen as important a testing ground for emotional intelligence as any Brechtian Lehrstücke (learning-plays). At the time of Brunsdon's writing, soaps were scheduled to coincide with tea-time, their episodic, fragmentary nature making them conducive to combining the execution of household chores with viewing. This connection to the sphere of reproductive immaterial labour made the form especially attractive to Zaman as a means of addressing the paternalistic ethos of the sphere of production. While the pleasures of cultural critique offered by the soap opera might pale before 'real' issues, Zaman's video, in oscillating between activism and cultural critique, performs a complex understanding of the pleasures of solidarity that paradoxically resonates with the hyperbolic fictional depictions of therapeutic self-exploitation in Beech's *Cannibals* and the related shorts *Well Being* and *Buried Alive.*

Some Women, Other Women and All the Bittermen does not simply advocate on behalf of the domestic workers' situation, but uses elliptical documentary footage of the workshop meetings between J4DW, Leeds Animation Workshop and art historian Charlesworth to question her own, and subsequent viewers', identification and distance from the domestic workers, as well as to interrupt the future propulsion of the soap narrative.[13] Whether moving between the six monitors in its initial installation or, as in my case, following the sequentiality of the single-screen version of the film, the shift between different registers of film-making becomes the means by which a transitional space of performative play opens up that complicates how the women are presented, avoiding the danger of appropriating representations of subaltern women as a point of resistance for a liberal Western mindset.[14]

As in the oscillation in Beech's *Cannibals* between the 'therapeutic potential of the groups' haptic experience' and how female empowerment is co-opted by neoliberal cognitive capitalism, Zaman's video also oscillates between exposing exploitative commodified values and an uncommodified therapeutic pleasure in group experience. This occurs in a number of sequences that show the pleasure in group work, both a dance sequence in episode four in which the women perform in front of their campaign banners to Shakira's *Waka Waka (This Time for Africa)* (2010), and a sequence showing members of J4DW learning animation techniques at the Leeds Animation Workshop. Zaman refers to the importance of the dance sequence for her own viewing of the women as subjects of pleasure rather than purely exploited workers: 'The scene provides a fuller picture of J4DW where women come together to experience joy communally as well as campaign and struggle to seek an end to modern slavery' (in Zaman and Guy, 2015). It is hard to garner precisely what is going on in the footage showing the domestic workers learning animation techniques. Much of this has to do with necessity and practicality, for example, point-of-view shots were not always possible as remaining invisible allows some of these women to continue working in the UK. However, Zaman deliberately included these more elliptical sequences in her edit 'to downplay the potential didacticism of the more overtly activist content', as well as to protect against positing the domestic workers as 'other or victim' (in Zaman and Guy, 2015). What began as a necessity becomes the formal aesthetics that keeps the video from being a campaign document in aid of the domestic workers' cause. The sequence of the animation workshop exudes the collective energy of being immersed in creative group activity akin to Bion's 'group-work mentality' (referred to in Chapter 7). These scenes also reference the history of radical filmmaking as exemplified by the Leeds Animation Workshop, thereby further alluding to the uncommodified value of another type of collective labour.[15]

But the notion of uncommodified therapeutic value is especially raised for me in the compelling sequences in the video in which the women's hands are framed in close-up as they continually rearrange the order of a series of Post-it notes on the workshop table. On the Post-it notes are written the words: 'home', 'faith', 'job', 'friends', 'security', and 'politics' – all terms loosely adapted from Abraham Maslow's theory of the 'hierarchy of needs' as proposed in his 1943 paper 'A Theory of Human Motivation'. This theory is usually visualized as a pyramidal diagram in which the more 'physiological' needs of food and shelter lie on the bottom with the individual attaining 'safety', 'belongingness' and 'love' as they move up the pyramid, before reaching the final achievements of 'esteem', 'self-actualization' and 'self-transcendence'. In both the women's adaptation and constant rearranging of these terms in the workshop discussions, which we overhear but cannot clearly determine, the items on the Post-its are transformed from hierarchical developmental needs to becoming co-dependent, horizontally distributive needs for *actualizing*, rather than merely sustaining, life.

It is interesting to read the horizontal reorganization of the Post-it notes in relation to Michel Feher's concept of 'self-appreciation' as discussed in his essay 'Self-Appreciation: Or, the Aspirations of Human Capital' (2009) in which he contrasts the free labourer of Fordism, i.e. the subject of unionized employment, and the new subjectivity of human capital. Rather than harking back to the liberal idea of unionized employment, premised as it is on an unsustainable model of world resources, Feher advises embracing the neoliberal condition to 'allow it to express aspirations and demands that its neoliberal promoters had neither intended nor foreseen' (2009: 25). While much of his argument is dependent on subjects who, unlike the domestic workers under current UK

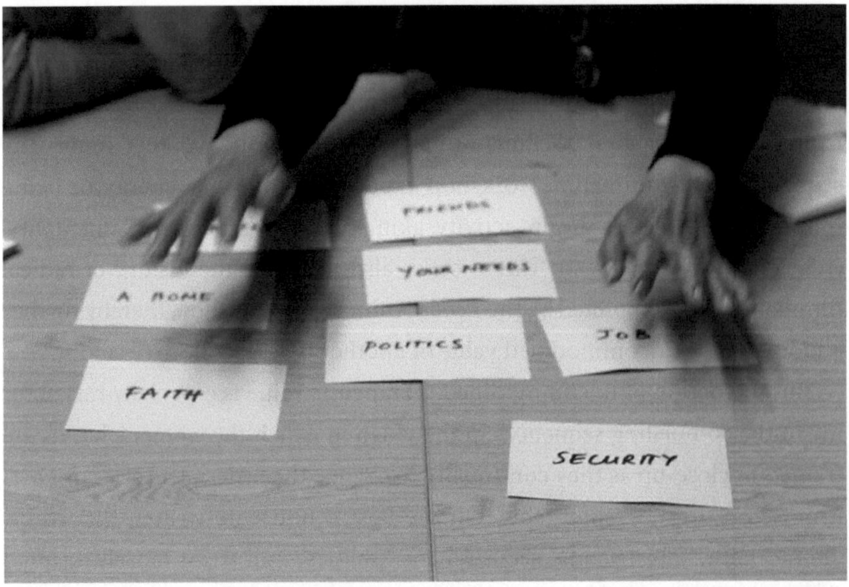

Figure 9.2 Rehana Zaman, *Some Women, Other Women and All the Bittermen*, 2014. Video still. Courtesy of the artist.

visa legislation, are free to move,[16] it nonetheless offers a thought-provoking way of thinking about the possibilities of uncommodified values suggested in both Beech's and Zaman's videos. For Feher, while capital eradicates the separation between the spheres of production and reproduction that existed in Fordist industrial labour and now extracts surplus value from the latter, this does not mean that it commodifies everything. For example, while the pleasures of group activity in *Cannibals*, both the collective exorcism of debilitating psychological behaviours and the cannibalistic implosion in the carnivalesque feast, are possibly recuperated for economic exchange relations, they need not be. They could instead be seen as investments in human capital, not in terms of the accruement of monetary profit, but in terms of collective well-being. Likewise, the list of needs on the Post-it notes in *Some Women, Other Women and All the Bittermen* propose a rethinking of Feher's notion of the 'required means for self-appreciation' (2009: 39). This was further brought home to me by Marissa Begonia, coordinator of J4DW (now The Voice of Domestic Workers) and featured in Zaman's video, at a panel event called 'On Social Reproduction' that took place at the ICA in London in

December 2015.[17] As well as discussing the campaign, Begonia also spoke about her self-esteem as the emotional and moral trainer for the child in her care as well as the pleasure and importance of dressing well when going to meet with MPs or attending public events on behalf of J4DW. So rather than esteem and self-actualization and/or self-appreciation being entities whose acquisition has to be postponed until physiological needs are met, they are intrinsic to life. Of course, domestic workers need a living wage and the right to move employer, but their 'transcendence' and 'joy' equally need to be acknowledged to prevent the subaltern being situated as a victim in need of rescue.

In both videos, therefore, the transpersonal therapeutic and empathic relations between female bodies are made palpable. Neoliberal capitalism engenders subjects who are supposed to be responsible for their own well-being, a subjectivity which is shown in *Cannibals* to walk a fine line between self-exploitative greed and potential solidarity. J4DW are self-organizing through necessity. They need legislation in order to enhance their capital so that they can live well despite the forced economic choices they have had to make in leaving their own families. Explored together, the videos underscore that we are unequally subjected to the same conditions of precarity that characterize forms of labour in neoliberal cognitive capitalism, yet the pleasure of group solidarity is a value that escapes commodification.

Sometime after writing this, I encountered feminist theorist Nancy Fraser's book *Fortunes of Feminism: From State-Managed Capitalism to Neoliberal Crisis* (2013) and found, to my surprise given my non-activist approach, that she also maintains that value and labour need to be separated. I would like to end this chapter by citing her thought-provoking conclusion. Rather than calling out for more forms of labour to be recognized as production, Fraser, somewhat echoing Federici, says that the crisis of neoliberalism offers feminists:

> the chance to break the spurious link between our critique of the family wage and flexible capitalism. Reclaiming our critique of androcentrism, feminists might militate for a form of life that decenters waged work and valorizes uncommodified activities, including, but not only, carework. Now performed largely by women, such activities should become valued components of a good life for everyone. (2013: 225–6)

10

Conclusion: Toxicity and self-care – two poles of pharmacological aesthetics

Steven Shaviro advocates an aesthetic of self-cultivation as a remedy to the insatiable and infinite desires of consumer capitalism 'where I stylize myself in order to market myself, to be an entrepreneur of myself, and to increase the value of my "human capital"' (2015: unpaginated). A notion of aesthetic self-cultivation might sound like an elitist, arcane set of practices[1] and in part it is, but in the last three chapters, I have been proffering the idea that it is a necessity for all despite social and economic obstacles. As Shaviro claims, '[i]n our world today, there is *already* enough accumulated wealth, and sufficiently advanced technology, for every human being to lead a life of leisure and self-cultivation' (2015: unpaginated). However, Shaviro's call for attention to be paid to everyday finite and transitory pleasures is dependent in part on a degree of economic comfort. In her study of aesthetic existence as a multimodal socially embedded corporeal endeavour, Monique Roelofs argues that the promise of the aesthetic is that it is available for everyone, yet its threat is that it is unequally available in an unjust system (2015). Nonetheless, she too concentrates on the inevitable ubiquity of 'aesthetic relationality', that is, the attachments to things that people adopt on a daily basis in order to cultivate pleasure in toxic situations (Roelofs, 2015: 8).[2]

As I explored in the previous chapter, while aesthetic self-cultivation depends on a certain level comfort and the satisfaction of needs such as food and shelter, this is not simply a middle-class ethos of individualism, but a communalist sensibility that everyone engages in regardless of whether it is economically enabled by the capitalist system. This is not to say that there should not be redistributive justice, but to recognize that even in conditions of extreme precarity, aesthetic self-cultivation, or what Foucault referred to as 'the care of the self' is a necessity, not a luxury. No art work can solve social problems, but in becoming an object we can 'use' aesthetically rather than instrumentally, my argument is that moving image artworks might operate as transitional spaces that maintain forms-of-life immune from cognitive capitalism's extraction of economic value from 'affective and aesthetic textures and experiences' (Smith in de Boever and Neidich, 2013: 39). This immunity is dependent on maintaining the imbrication of the toxic and the curative in order to avoid subjection to prevailing ideologies that use the rhetoric of remedy to deny underlying poisons or threats. In this concluding chapter, I want to briefly explore this imbrication in relation to self-care and/as resistance.

I first started researching this book in 2014. As I come to the end of the project, there has been a burgeoning of overtly therapeutic thematics in contemporary artists' work and in art venues. This is due in part to the conditions of neoliberal capitalism in which a decrease in public funding has led to an increased demand for accountability. Part of this involves questioning art's purpose in a social climate of enforced poverty due to, what I would call, the technique of austerity. By contrast to my focus on pharmacological therapeutic aesthetics in which the toxic and the curative are mutually imbricated and at play, much of this burgeoning of the therapeutic focuses on instrumentalizing art either to politicize personal illness[3] or to use it to remedy the effects of social discrimination.[4] Much of it coalesces around the term 'self-care', which is fast becoming a commoditized value in the art world of cognitive capitalism rather than relating to the transvaluation of values implicit in Foucault's 'the care of the self' that I referred to in Chapter 8. In the guise of the former, self-care functions as a purely positive act that responds to the psychopathologies of 'the achievement society', adding value to that society by reactively subscribing to its mores. For example, I am stressed therefore I will take time out for a trip to the spa or a yoga retreat – I can afford this luxury if I am in gainful employment and it will enable me to work more productively, which in turn will enable me to afford, and need, more such treatments. However, in work by some artists of colour, e.g. Simone Leigh and Carolyn Lazard, the kinds of illnesses and pathologies that are being cared for, whether in group or solo works, are not purely psychological or biological but bound up in the legacies of colonialism and the techniques of racism and classism which has meant that swathes of society do not even get a look-in in 'the achievement society'. In this context, self-care, to cite the much often cited Audre Lorde, 'is not self-indulgence, it is self-preservation, and that is an act of political warfare' (1988: 130).[5] However, remaining within the parameters of my pharmacological argument, I want to briefly reorient self-care in relation to my encounter with another film by Zaman, *Sharla Shabana Sojourner Selena* (2016), in which I propose that the productive simultaneity of the reparative and the destructive that characterizes transitional space is acted out. Rather than seeking to redeem past traumas and move into a future wholeness, this simultaneity attends to 'the moment of disturbance before form provides an anchor' (Berlant in Berlant and Povinelli, 2014). Zaman's use of performativity in *Sharla Shabana Sojourner Selena* pivots on this moment of disturbance, the film's therapeutic aesthetics being to reorient and refashion, but not cure, the toxicities of sexism and racism. However, before I go on to look at the film, I want to adumbrate the relation between self-care and toxicity as two extremes on either side of the pharmacological passage between opposites. My purpose here is to suggest why it is desirable that a pharmacological therapeutic aesthetics keeps the toxic side of the equation in play.

First to self-care. Self-care has a long history evolving from feminist and collective political consciousness-raising of the 1960s and 1970s, in which it figures as a tool of self-healing to resist oppression and discrimination. However, this latter modality and Foucault's notion of 'the care of the self' involving philosophical examination, as well as aesthetic practices of bodily maintenance that I referred to in Chapter 8, are currently subsumed by consumer capitalism and its emphasis on individualism. For example, the internet movement #selfcare, fashioned around 2016, mainly advocates indulgence in luxury treats combined with mindfulness techniques such as mediation, yoga and even the gym, all considered modes of cognitive and emotional repair that contribute to healthier bodies that can remain resilient in a neoliberal economy of incessant competition and precarity.[6] The term 'self-care' has also become a diagnostic label linked to austerity politics – people are encouraged to take care of themselves by exercising and eating well so as not to be a burden on stripped back medical and social services, yet paradoxically statistics show increases in anxiety, depression, ADHD and chronic fatigue (https://www.mentalhealth.org.uk/publications/fundamental-facts-about-mental-health, 2016). Although specific to the UK, such statistics are not unique to it, aligning as they do with philosophical speculation by Stiegler, Berardi, Shaviro and Han that adumbrate these symptoms as reactions to the general insecurity, precarity and marketization of values promulgated in and by neoliberal cognitive capitalism. In an article in *The New Yorker*, 'The Politics of Conspicuous Displays of Self-Care', Jordan Kisner jauntily writes that '"Self-care" rose as a collective social practice in 2016 alongside national stress levels' (2017). According to Kisner, the term has a particular resonance in the American lexicon that links it to self-reliance, both notions stemming from the puritanical values of self-improvement and self-examination or what Stanley Cavell refers to as 'the self-cultivating individual' (2017). This idea links with Lauren Berlant's thesis in *Cruel Optimism* that, while the American dream was/is an organizing fantasy of progress and achievement that excludes swathes of the American population, its fantasy of self-cultivation may nonetheless be invested in by those it excludes, albeit to damaging effect given the social and economic obstacles to their flourishing. In this light, self-care, if it is to have any pharmacological therapeutic value, needs to be repoliticized as an act of self-preservation and resistance rather than a lifestyle choice. As Kisner describes it, self-care was 'repopularized in the seventies and eighties by people of color and queer communities—this time as a gesture of defiance' (2017). Going on to cite Lorde's aforementioned rallying cry, Kisner asserts: 'In this formulation, self-care was no longer a litmus test for social equality; it was a way to insist to a violent and oppressive culture that you mattered, that you were worthy of care' (2017).[7]

A similar article by Arwa Mahdawi in the UK newspaper *The Guardian*, also in 2017, further underscores the contrast between self-care as a radical act of survival and self-care as an individualized response to the pathologies of cognitive capitalism such as burnout and stress from aspirational over-achievement. As Mahdawi says:

> It's nice to think that our bubble baths and personal time might have a larger political purpose ('Um, Foucault! I'm not *just* bingeing Netflix – I'm engaging in Platonic political philosophy in order to better serve others!'), but more often than not, our acts of self-care are simply acts of privilege. (2017)

As opposed to this, Kisner proposes that for disenfranchised persons, self-care is resistance (2017).

There is no denying that acts of self-care as self-cultivation can be empowering; however, in 'Toxic Assemblages, Queer Socialities: A Dialogue of Mutual Poisoning' (2013), Antke Engel and Renate Lorenz propose appropriating toxicity, not self-care, as resistance. I can hear accusations of white privilege as I write this sentence, but as Engel and Lorenz conceive it, there is a rationale to playing with the toxic that is not exclusive to those who are perceived as having privilege in white supremacist patriarchy. Engel's and Lorenz's view of toxicity also counters Stiegler's philosophically moral premise in which care as a good is premised on the cultivation of civility, whereas bad care channels attention to objects that are impermanent and distracting, i.e. unmindful.

Engel and Lorenz focus on *Toxic* (2012), an installation that Lorenz made with Pauline Boudry.[8] As they describe it, the installation includes a thirteen-minute film shot on 16mm and featuring drag queens Werner Hirsch, who stars as a punk, and Ginger Brooks Takahashi, as well as a vitrine with fifteen photographs of so-called pédérastes taken in bourgeois commercial photographic studios in the early 1870s before the birth of the mug shot. Engel and Lorenz discuss how, both at the level of its materiality and at the level of representation, photographic film and digital production depend on toxicity: in the first instance, in relation to chemicals; and, in the latter instance, in relation to how photography was used in late nineteenth-century mug-shots as a tool of racialization and 'othering' that documented and categorized minorities according to a colonial and/or imperial gaze. However, for Engel and Lorenz such images can also engender meanings and resonances other than the stereotypical categorizing and exclusionary policies of colonial and psychiatric photography. They claim that when it comes to these images that were used as models for mug-shots 'neither the effects nor the critical dosage is predictable' (2013). Casting those pictured in the mug-shots as 'queer', Engel and Lorenz pose what for me is a crucial pharmacological question: 'if one longs for recognition and the inclusion of differences and singularities, but does not believe in or agree to being subsumed within neoliberal pluralism, how can one resist?' (2013). As a strategy of enabling singularity, but resisting hegemony, they deploy the notion of toxicity as a kind of psycho-social performativity which would entail incorporating and acting out the very toxicity that society accuses you of. This performative process involves what they call, riffing off Deleuze's and Guattari's philosophy of becoming, a '*becoming-indigestible*', a notion which

> underlines the paradoxical moment of being incorporated, yet not built into the system. It refers to the idea of toxicity, since it implies remaining non-assimilable. [...] The toxic—resisting being digested and split up into useful parts that can be integrated into the system—turns out to be a means of either changing or, maybe, destroying the system from within. (2013)

In terms of aesthetic practices, this would involve an appropriation of imagery considered toxic by the mainstream in order to show how 'subjectivities developing from processes of intoxication may decide to function as toxic themselves rather than seeking detoxification' (Engel and Lorenz, 2013). Rather than the toxic scapegoat seeking entry into a community by shedding its toxicity and adapting to that society, the scapegoat, which is also another meaning of the term 'pharmakon', appropriates toxicity as a means of self-determination or cultivation. This echoes Butler's argument in *Excitable Speech* (1997), in which she advocates the reclaiming of injurious speech by groups and identities towards whom such speech is directed in acts of racial and sexual scapegoating and stereotyping, e.g. the re-appropriation of terms such as 'queer' by the communities towards whom the term was directed as a term of abuse. In the film *Toxic*, Hirsch voices all the toxic slurs she can think of, this sounding aloud being an act of both incorporation and exorcism. In this act, subjectivities that are seen as a problem for the socius perform their toxic markers of discrimination without seeking to restore them to pool of social well-being, as the latter would serve to pacify the (neo)liberal consciousness that it speaks to and includes plurality.[9] Instead, Engels and Lorenz ask what dosages (of images) might enable toxicity to develop 'pleasurable, enabling, surprising, and curative effects' (2013). In other words, how might technologies that poison and hurt also cure and empower? But crucially, this cure needs to retain its partially indigestible, toxic aspect so as to enable socialities that would not be formed 'by healthy, sane, and self-same bodies claiming wholeness, autonomy, and control' (Engels and Lorenz, 2013).

The combination of the curative and the unassimilable in Engel's and Lorenz's concept of toxicity has parallels with Stiegler's deconstructive argument of the pharmakon as both poison and cure. However, Engel's and

Lorenz's use of toxicity to queer the assimilative aspect of cure raises the question of what it might mean for subjects who have been classed as toxic to take care of themselves in environments that do not take care of them. My question is how a moving image artwork might function as a transitional space in which speech and gestural acts deflect toxicity without denying its existence. While Stiegler (2013a) sees transitional space as a prototype of a desire-based economy of pleasure, whereby pleasure derives from having the time to attend to things, to contemplate and to take care of objects, nonetheless a certain violence and disequilibrium are necessarily involved in the cultivation of the world. Damage and repair have to be thought in tandem. Zaman's *Sharla Shabana Sojourner Selena* complicates ideas of self-care as simply reactive or transformative. While the film's performativity refuses to eradicate the toxicity of injury and damage, unlike Engel's and Lorenz's toxic homeopathy, Zaman's 'moment of disturbance before form provides an anchor' is more open to the curative pole of the pharmakon, which is ultimately the note on which I wish to end this book.

Sharla Shabana Sojourner Selena comprises a series of performance-to-camera vignettes by six actresses, who recount partly scripted, partly improvised experiences of racism and sexism, most of which are obliquely recounted as micro-aggressions whose 'actants' are not easy to identify as victims or aggressors. These sequences, shot against a stark studio location, are interposed with sequences shot in 'Acacia', a hair and beauty salon. The film opens with a sequence shot in this site of self-care treatments in which three of the actresses recite a script cut-up and adapted from a Bion case study in *Experiences in Groups* (1961). Their dialogue consists of a series of non sequiturs that are relayed between them, beginning with, 'I'm unwell ... I was standing in a queue and nearly passed out ... at least you weren't standing ... I was sitting quietly at home' and so forth. For Zaman, the dialogue epitomizes how individuals in groups often converse at cross purposes to one another, an idea Bion discusses in terms of how a certain type of 'group mentality' can allow individual frustrations to be expressed anonymously. (See Chapter 7 for more specific detail on Bion's theories of groups.) As the film proceeds, the talking head vignettes are intercut with close-ups of the beauty treatments – pedicures, nail-painting and attaching false eyelashes. One mixed heritage woman recounts a scenario in a restaurant in which her boyfriend was heroically celebrated by a couple after he saved the female partner from choking while she was ignored. Another black woman recounts how she was not allowed to take up a position of leadership within her church because of her gender, while another woman of colour describes an incident of racial discrimination at an audition that resulted in her being rejected for a part. Part of the inspiration for the film was Zaman's participation on a panel following a screening of experimental filmmaker Chick Strand's *Soft Fiction* (1979) at Tate Modern in 2015 in which the panel's raising the question of the absence of 'women of colour' in Strand's film was dismissed as irrelevant by some of the audience who wanted to situate her purely in the history of American experimental film.[10] Zaman wanted to complicate this picture by only casting 'women of colour' in her film, not simply to reverse racial categorization but to performatively complicate it.

While Zaman has said that she was thinking about therapy in making the film, for me, its therapeutic aesthetics has less to do with a commonsense notion of therapy and healing than with the way the women's monologues entice viewers to move beyond racialized categorization into a more open, yet critical, space of play. The women's performances are not straightforwardly confessional acts, but (re)enactments that oscillate between reciting and recalling, teasing and accusing, there being an extraordinary slippage in the film's enunciative voice as to who is speaking and who is being addressed. For example, the second performance-to-camera features a young black actress who claims that she has spent all her time trying to be accepted into the university by reading dead white men's texts and yet she is still excluded. This statement can easily be read in the context of racist forms of micro-aggression endemic to the power structures of UK universities, but the actress' recitation of her lines also conveyed a performative linguistic structure that opened up the scenario to being potentially, if partially, inhabited by others who might not necessarily identify as a 'woman of colour'. While the performative nature of her statement is underscored towards the end of the film by its almost work-for-word repetition by another of the actresses, her words hit me as partly describing my own interpellation by the university as a white woman whose relation to imperial and colonial power is defined by a long history of transgenerational and enforced migration. I found myself moving between inhabiting the actress' speech act and being excluded from it, the enunciative relay and repetition of her speech act engendering a space in which a circumnavigation of the parameters of racism and sexism could take place without creating diametrically opposed positions between victims and perpetrators. It engendered a space in which on- and off-screen actors might move with at least enough ambulation to explore partial positionalities and identifications beyond the optics that mark the bodies of women of colour as carriers of otherness in 'white supremacist capitalistic patriarchy' (hooks in Patierno et al., 1997: 7).[11] This performative relay of experience was simultaneously being deconstructed by the camera – the camera wavers up, down and across cropped torsos, especially focusing on hand gestures rather than remaining statically fixed on the speaking bodies. In this dual interplay, while the toxic damage of racism and sexism remains in play, it is relayed across a spectrum that unhinges it from individual trauma. What I am getting at here is the possibility of a performative therapeutics of the image in which speech acts operate to defy projections of what is expected of an individual based on socially prescribed identitarian categories or capture within the visual field of colonial and patriarchal technologies. The performative therapeutics enacted by *Sharla Shabana Sojourner Selena* opened up a space in which pain, anger, desire and joy simultaneously reverberated within the (re)enactments of scripted and improvised experiences punctuated by shots of cropped body parts – nails and eyelids – being treated with care and the sound of laughter.

This could be conceptualized in a number of ways, but sticking with performativity, I want to reiterate Butler's hopeful idea that the strategy of engaging in performative speech acts in ritualistic contexts might enable the re-signification of injurious incidents or speech. In this, Butler was inspired by Derrida's notion of the instability of the sign in his essay 'Signature Event Context' ([1972] 1988). However, as Diana Taylor summarizes it, Derrida's emphasis on the importance of citationality and iterability in the event of speech begs the question of 'whether a performative statement [could] succeed if its formulation did not repeat a "coded" or iterable statement' (Taylor, 2003: 5). For Taylor, Butler subsumes 'subjectivity and cultural agency into normative discursive practice' (6) rather than remaining with Austin's consideration of language as something that acts. While Butler's notion of performativity is more complex than this, nonetheless it has often been criticized for not offering a more definitive transformative politics, as its emphasis on the repetition of social norms risks the reproduction of the same. Taylor turns to other strands of performance studies that can help in rethinking the transformative moment in the present rather than as a future yet to come. She points out that in both the dramaturgical tradition of anthropology (Victor Turner, Clifford Geertz and Erving Goffman) and the linguistic stream of anthropologists influenced by Austin (Gregory Bateson, Richard Bauman and Michele Rosaldo), stress is placed on 'the creativity at play in the use of language, as speakers and their audiences worked together to produce successful verbal performances' (Taylor, 2003: 7). Both traditions maintained 'the creativity in the everyday life of other people, ways of using language that were resourceful, specific and "authentic"' (7). As I mentioned from the outset, performativity is always both linguistic and dramaturgical (Sedgwick, 2003), though the latter aspect has garnered less attention in contemporary art theory. As both linguistic and dramaturgical, the performativity of therapeutic aesthetics can regenerate speech and gestural acts as shared and disseminated in the ritualistic (transitional) spaces of moving image artworks such as *Sharla Shabana Sojourner Selena*.[12]

Immersing its viewers in close-up shots that focus attention on feet being pumiced, eyes being treated and nails being painted by hands whose fingernails

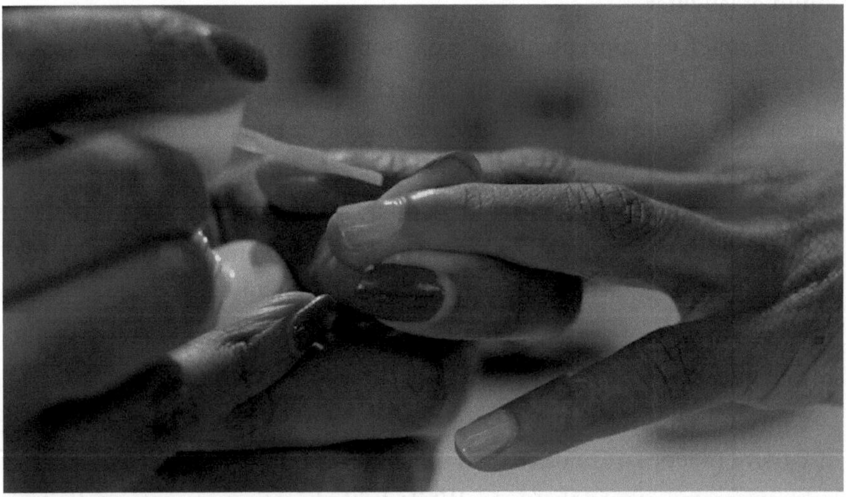

Figure 10.1 Rehana Zaman, *Sharla Shabana Sojourner Selena*, 2016. Video still. Courtesy of the artist.

are always coated in metallic red varnish, the film suggests that while the clients swop places, the 'aesthetician', another name for a beauty therapist, is the same person. However, the rhythm of the bodily gestures in tandem with the tinny pop music in the background implies mutual enjoyment. While the reality is that the women who work in these salons are often exploited for their labour and therefore in an economically subservient relation to their clients, this is not the story the film's images tell. And neither does it fit neatly into the narrative of using beauty therapy as an indulgent mode of self-care. The underlying economies of the salon as a service industry notwithstanding, the film portrays an intimate exchange of pleasure and well-being between women of colour, asymmetry here not excluding mutuality.[13] These gestures become acts of sensual survivance, to appropriate Berlant's term, that resist the co-option of beauty treatments as either luxury indulgences to be frowned upon or necessary luxuries to defend against the toxic environment of neoliberal cognitive capitalism. In this ritualistic transitional space, a pleasurable giving and receiving of care divorced from ownership is intimated. Whose feet? Whose hands? The final shot hones in on a cotton face pad. A hand enters the frame and scars it with red polish, the excess residue on a nail brush, the humour of the sequence underlining the material toxicities of the beauty salon as well as their joyful applications.

Conclusion

For subjects who are positioned differently in relation to the status quo, the aesthetics of everyday life is the very sphere in which acts of micro-resistance occur in a non-reifiable way, e.g. the pleasure one might get from sitting in a communal garden.[14] However, the performative acts of micro-resistance I have been looking at in artists' moving image works are inherently pharmacological, whereas sitting in a communal garden could be seen as a more commonsensically therapeutic act that momentarily eradicates toxicity. Though, on the other hand, such acts are also performative to the extent that they need to be continually repeated to manage toxicity. As long as they are not merely socially prescribed, people do extract their own forms of well-being from such everyday practices of aesthetic self-cultivation despite the exclusions encountered and damage executed in and by neoliberal capitalism. In my argument, the beauty salon in *Sharla Shabana Sojourner Selena* is envisioned less as a space where one recharges one's batteries to re-engage in the sphere of production and 'the achievement society', but more a space and time akin to Berlant's notion of survivance as a pleasurable hanging out in the impasse of the present:

> the impasse is a stretch of time in which one moves around with a sense that the world is at once intensely present and enigmatic, such that the activity of living demands both a wandering absorptive awareness and a hypervigilance that collects material that might help to clarify things, maintain one's sea legs, and coordinate the standard melodramatic crises with those processes that have not yet found their genre of event. (2011: 4)

In this temporality, flourishing is created from the shards of fractured experience without projecting a concept of the future. Berlant refers to this temporality as a de-dramatized 'recasting [of] the traumatic event into an ordinary intensity' (2011: 86).

In the moving image artworks assembled in this book, I have been interested in their use of various performative techniques that mimic traumatic experiential conditions. Beginning with case studies that staged or documented the pharmacological performativity of technology in relation to PTSD, I traced how the poisonous aspects of homeopathic mimicry came to the fore in Farocki's *Serious Games* without however reneging on its curative potential. I also looked at how in Fast's invented narratives revolving around PTSD, trauma was displaced to such an extent that viewers might be seduced to engage in stories they would ordinarily recoil from, the work providing a kind of inoculating effect to enable this. Continuing to diagnose the mores and psychopathologies of cognitive capitalism, I looked to Gilligan's speculative fictions for a topographic and pedagogical mapping of affective and cognitive subjectification and her exploration of the potential of a new collective subjectivity as a remedy to the latter. Following the implosion of this potential in her work, I examined its impossibility as long as identitarian subjects are in thrall to political leaders as acted out in Laser's *Primal Speech*. However, 'using' Laser's work as a transitional object led me to shift from a critical diagnosis of the psychopathologies of cognitive and neoliberal capitalism to more proximity to the curative dimension of the pharmacological that nonetheless suspends the goal of healing as wholeness. Rather, as demonstrated in Ledare's staged workshops based on the Tavistock Institute's theories of group dynamics as well as the use of Method acting training in Wearing's *Self Made*, self-cultivation is inherently fraught with toxicity. Acknowledging this allows for the ambivalence and unpredictability of singularity, an ethos that pervades Fox's *The* O *Show* in which 'exposure therapy' as a means of self-determination that is not reducible to capital is validated. Beech's and Zaman's films opened up issues of gender and race in relation to affective labour as well as complicating what might be deemed self-appreciation by and for whom. In this shift from the diagnostic to the creativity of the performative, I have moved far from my launching pad, i.e. Stiegler's notion of the pharmacological, and more towards the Berardian idea of art as a kind of treatment 'a kind of psychotherapy that might lead us towards the type of creation that can resist the psychological implosion wrought by our interface with capitalism' (Berardi in Zepke, 2012: 221). However, rather than this being a goal, my argument is that this art treatment transmits the pleasures of scepticism as well as the potential of provisional healing. This is a 'good enough' therapeutic in which protagonists can use their performative selves as transitional objects that enable the toxic and the curative to be thought in tandem with one another rather than one side being celebrated as a positive value while the other is suppressed or denied.

My shift in emphasis in this book from homeopathic mimicry as a form of resistance to artworks that adopt the self-cultivation required for liveable lives resonates with the temporality of what Berlant calls 'living on' past the event of implosion (2011: 70). It is a temporality oriented to the present tense rather than Stiegler's future-oriented philosophy or Shaviro's catastrophic model of implosion. 'Living on' is not mere survival but is linked, for Berlant, to Henri Lefebvre's rhythmanalysis as 'the mode of enacting life through habituated gestures that stretch the present out so that enjoyment is possible, a kind of autopoetic proprioceptive dressage' (2011: 63). This sense of well-being 'that spreads out for a moment' (Berlant, 2011: 117) is importantly distinct from the one that governmental bodies exhort us to achieve as responsible agents for our own mental health and welfare, an exhortation in which aesthetic practices, including visiting galleries and museums, are prescribed as cures for distress. The problem with the latter is that it denies both the reality and creativity of traumatic/toxic experience and integrates it into a redemptive narrative of social healing. Bersani's warning in the 1990s that 'the catastrophes of history matter much less if they are somehow compensated for in art, and art itself gets reduced to a kind of superior patching function' (9) is newly prescient. The instrumentalization of art transforms it into a form of compensation that is deemed to repair 'inherently damaged or valueless experience' (Bersani, 1990: 1). By contrast, performativity, in the linguistic and theatrical sense, keeps open the negotiation of experience and history, so that self-care is not a cure for trauma or psychopathological disorders, but an aesthetic *instituting* of spaces in which the parameters of poison and cure can be played with. This is not a panacea for social ills, but a constant process of reformulation in which '*we pay attention* to what takes shape from within the disturbances of relationality' (Berlant in Berlant and Povinelli, 2014). I confess that I have used moving image artworks in this way, both to inoculate me against the shocks of everyday life[15] and to keep me alert to those disturbances in which toxicity remains generative and unassimilated. As a pharmakon, the moving image artwork can act as a homeopathic mimicry of the disabling symptoms that are contagiously generated in the capitalist affectsphere (Berlant, 2011), but, in so doing, it also reaches beyond them to find the pleasures hidden by the strangleholds of world-homogenizing systems. As a conflictual form of treatment, the transitional spaces modelled by the moving image artworks assembled here invite a 'use' of the object that imagines ways of being otherwise.

Notes

Chapter 1

1 In struggling with the counterintuitive notion of therapeutic aesthetics as both critical and affirmative of the instrumentalization of art in cognitive capitalism, I was comforted to read Tina M. Campt's claim in *Listening to Images* that her arguments emerge from 'the endlessly generative space of the counterintuitive' (2017: 6).

2 Aesthetics as a branch of Western philosophy has a long history from its 'invention' in 1735 by Alexander Gottlieb Baumgarten and development by Immanuel Kant in his *Critique of Judgment* (1790).

3 This is notwithstanding the so-called return to beauty by critics such as Dave Hickey in the 1990s. For a potted history of the aesthetic and its social transmogrification, see Jill Bennett's book in the *RaRa* series *Practical Aesthetics: Events, Affect and Art after 9/11*, London and New York: I.B. Tauris, 2012.

4 The National Alliance for Arts Health and Wellbeing merged with The National Alliance for Museums, Health & Wellbeing to become The Culture, Health and Wellbeing Alliance in 2018.

5 Furedi's identification of 'a shift from social equality to equality of esteem' (2004: 169) is echoed by Ecclestone and Hayes (2009), who argue that the emergence of 'emotional well-being into political and professional thinking moves mental health work from a marginal activity into mainstream education and welfare services' (17). For a similar account of this shift in the United States, see James Nolan (1998).

6 Byung-Chul Han also uses these terms to classify the symptoms of the 'achievement society' in his short book *The Burnout Society* (2015).

7 For a pop cultural account of viewing art as a mode of therapy see A. de Botton and J. Armstrong, *Art as Therapy* (2016).

8 Terranova refers to the consistent use of the term 'cognitive capitalism' by Yann Moulier Boutang (2011) and others such as Carlo Vercellone, while Jodi Dean, Franco Berardi, Andrea Fumagalli and Cristina Morini, and David Harvey respectively deploy the other terms. She also refers to Vercellone's definition of

cognitive capitalism as defining the new paradigm of work in which surplus value is extracted from intellectual, immaterial and relational forms of living labour (Terranova in Neidich, 2013: 47).

9 See Ewa Hess and Hennric Jokeit, 'Neurocapitalism', at https://www.opendemocracy.net/en/neurocapitalism/ (accessed 29 July 2019), for an engaging account of the dynamic relation between capitalism and neuroscience.

10 Stiegler generally refers to consumerist capitalism.

11 Wilson does not take a stand for or against antidepressants, arguing instead that if we knew that there was no way of extracting the good from the bad, this might lead to a different form of governance and distribution of drugs. Her theoretical argument about the necessity of maintaining the edge between the entanglement of both good and bad deploys Melanie Klein's theories of reparation as well as Eve Kosofsky Sedgwick's notion of reparative and paranoid criticism, which I shall also refer to in later chapters.

12 While Butler's idea has been criticized for not offering a definitive pathway towards a transformative politics, her idea that such a transformation is possible via the repetition of social ritual continues to inspire artists and writers. In appending performativity to the artists' moving image case studies I explore, I am claiming that while not offering 'talking cures', they nonetheless perform a conflictual mitigation of the toxic effects of neoliberalism, their presentations of loosely (per)formed communities challenging, while participating in, therapeutic discourses of well-being and health.

13 This inoculation effect relates to Walter Benjamin's idea that film technology can enable audiences to deal with the shocks of modern life, not by simply lulling them into a collective stupor, but by replicating its shock effects, the survival of which enables coping with such events in everyday life. This can be extended to on-screen characters also, Benjamin's notion being that the film apparatus possesses a neuro-physiological process or energy that mediates between internal and external and human and non-human worlds.

14 See Toscano and Kinkle's *Cartographies of the Absolute* (2015: 47) for a brief account of Gilligan's *Crisis in the Credit System* (2008) in this light.

15 In Guattari's therapeutic aesthetics 'the only acceptable finality of human activity is the production of a subjectivity that is auto-enriching its relation to the world in a continuous fashion' (Guattari, 1995: 21).

16 'Survivance' is a term used in Indigenous Studies. It means more than mere survival and is rather a way of life that nourishes. See http://survivance.org/acts-of-survivance/, accessed 22 November 2019. The term is used by Elizabeth E. Povinelli in relation to the films of the Karrabing Film Collective.

Chapter 2

1 For another view of immanent critique in relation to Harun Farocki, see Nicole Brenez's 'Harun Farocki and the Romantic Genesis of the Principle of Visual Critique' in Ehmann and Eshun (eds.), 2010.

2 Hauser and Wirth press release, 2015. https://www.hauserwirth.com/hauser-wirth-exhibitions/5154-pipilotti-rist-worry-will-vanish, accessed 27 March 2019.

3 The soundtrack was a collaboration with artist and musician Anders Guggisberg.

4 Beller is alluding to Guy Debord's indictment of the socially divisive effects of capitalism in *The Society of the Spectacle* (1967), in which he defined spectacle not as 'a collection of images, but a social relation among people mediated by images' (Beller, 2006: 211). Beller describes spectacle as the enemy: 'today there is an almost palpable integument overlaying society [that] can no longer properly be described as "ideology" (since ideology is a concept welded to a narrative and therefore a quasi-historical core) but is more adequately denoted by the term "spectacle"' (2006: 214).

5 While the key reference for rhythmanalysis is of course Henri Lefebvre (2004), my concluding chapter will return to it via Lauren Berlant's appropriation of it in relation to modes of pleasurable survivance in restricted circumstances (2011).

6 While Stiegler moves in the direction of digital media, recent literature on psychoanalysis and televisual media also refers to media objects as transitional phenomena by and through which users/viewers work through various psychic fantasies and problems in life-enhancing ways. See Bainbridge, Ward and Yates (eds.), 2014.

7 Buck-Morss argues that the original development of aesthetics was in line with the development of the human sensorium in eighteenth-century philosophy. They parted ways in the nineteenth century, only to come together again in the twentieth century in relation to a changing conception of the brain as less a biological organ but more part of a nervous system that is open to and in a dynamic relation to the world environment.

8 Shaviro's other examples include mainstream films: Mark Neveldine and Brian Taylor's *Gamer* (2009); Olivier Assayas' *Boarding Gate* and Richard Kelly's *Southland Tales*, both from 2007.

Chapter 3

1 As Volker Pantenburg states: 'what Farocki discovered in the 80s as one of the cornerstones of his observational cinema was that the kinds of performance and

performativity that Brecht utilized to construct new forms of theatre have also long permeated the actual fabric of society's institutions and rituals' (Pantenburg in Balsom and Peleg (eds.), *Documentary across Disciplines*, Berlin: Haus der Kulturen der Welt: 2016), p.156.

2 Celis Bueno is specifically referring to Farocki's work in the 2000s and his notion of 'operational images', i.e. images that are produced by machines. While the images in *How to Live in the FRG* are documentary, they nonetheless function in the film in an automatic non-teleological manner. Farocki's 'immanent critique' is also discussed by Nicole Brenez in her essay 'Harun Farocki and the Romantic Genesis of the Principle of Visual Critique', in Ehmann and Eshun (2009, pp.128–42).

3 Although my use of the term 'subjectivation' stems directly from Lazzarato and Félix Guattari, they are referencing Michel Foucault's concept which denotes the intentional work of an individual on itself in order to subject itself to a set of moral recommendations for conduct and, as a result of this 'subjectivation', or self-forming activity, constitute its own ethics. I am using this more generally to mean, paraphrasing Stiegler, knowledge of how-to-live. Foucault's ethics are elaborated in *The Use of Pleasure* and *The Care of the Self*. For more information, see https://www.iep.utm.edu/fouc-eth/, accessed 27 February 2020.

4 In his introduction to his very informative interview with Stiegler, Lemmons further summarizes this, stating that in 'today's service economies, consumers are "discharged" of the burden as well as the responsibility of shaping their own lives and are reduced to units of buying power controlled by marketing techniques', a situation that replaces know-how with 'preformatted and standardized "lifestyles" fabricated and marketed on a worldwide scale by global corporations exclusively driven by profit' (Lemmens, 2011: 33).

5 Markham is specifically referring to how viewers might relate to news media reportage, not as a call to action or a dismissal of tragic events.

6 For a detailed historical account of this history, see Sally Alexander's essay 'D.W. Winnicott and the social democratic vision', in Matt ffytche and Daniel Pick (eds.), *Psychoanalysis in the Age of Totalitarianism* (Abingdon and New York: Routledge, 2016), pp.114–30.

7 See Peter Osborne's essay 'Distracted Reception: Time, Art and Technology', in *Time Zones: Recent Film and Video,* Jessica Morgan and Gregor Muir (eds.) (London: Tate, 2004), pp.66–75, as well as Pasi Väliaho's discussion of Farocki in *Biopolitical Screens: Image, Power, and the Neoliberal Brain* (Cambridge, MA: MIT Press Leonardo, 2014).

8 In fact, in the essay 'Organology of Dreams and Archi-Cinema' (2013b), Stiegler refers to this eruption as a traumatype harking back to the deferred time of Freudian trauma as an event in the past whose mnemic traces erupt into a newly significant context in the present.

9 One of the most prominent illnesses claimed today is post-traumatic stress disorder, an illness which only entered the *DSM* in 1980. Initially used to describe symptoms experienced by war veterans, it is increasingly being used to describe all manner of stress-related illnesses from anorexia to panic attacks.

10 The full title being Immersive Infantry Trainer and Advanced Simulator Combat Operations and Training. See *Killer Images* (2012), p.66.

11 According to Sara Brady, citing the Rand corporation website, one in five veterans of Iraq and Afghanistan war suffers from PTSD characterized by flashbacks and nightmares lasting more than a month (Brady, 2012: 97).

12 Leys refers to the work of neuropsychologist Bessel von der Kolk, amongst others, who maintains that traumatic memories are stored intact in the brain and that their retrieval and conscious recall enable their exorcism. For Leys this is a dubious notion.

13 For an in-depth account of the design of VRET, see Marisa Renee Brandt's unpublished PhD thesis 'War, Trauma, and Technologies of the Self: The Making of Virtual Reality Exposure Therapy' (2013) UC San Diego, https://escholarship.org/content/qt6698t67t/qt6698t67t.pdf, accessed 6 September 2019.

14 This technique is called 'soft montage'. Nicole Brenez refers to this as 'comparativism through juxtaposition and putting into series, which transfer to space the temporal principle inherent to the intermittence of film frames in cinema' (in Ehmann and Eshun, 2009: 129).

15 For another approach to immunity and capitalist structures, see Esposito (2013).

16 This article features a case study of a veteran with chronic PTSD who was able to tolerate exposure to pictures serving as triggers for traumatic memories that he had greatly suppressed and avoided talking about.

17 In the 1990s, Cathy Caruth introduced the notion that trauma is performative; i.e. it acts rather than represents (Leys, 2000: 267). Caruth's approach gains a new credence in relation to neurobiological ideas about the modularity, flexibility and autonomy of the brain in illnesses such as trauma from an accident and dementia (Malabou, *The New Wounded: From Neurosis to Brain Damage*, 2012) that disconnect the relation between trauma and repression and consider it instead as a psychosomatic phenomenon open to technological

image treatments. It is perhaps notable that VR games are being developed as treatments for dementia sufferers.

18 For information on this artwork, see Pugh (2016).

19 Email to author, 16 August 2019.

Chapter 4

1 Subsequently the museum purchased the work as part of its collection.

2 See Cathy Caruth, *Unclaimed Experience: Trauma, Narrative, and History* (Baltimore and London: Johns Hopkins University Press, 1996).

3 My notes from Judith Butler's presentation at the event 'Enduring and Broken Time–Judith Butler and Lisa Baraitser' at Birkbeck University on 14 June 2018.

4 I am basing my description of the installation on my encounter with it at Tate Modern, London in 2013 as part of the museum's changing displays.

5 Fast admits the stress of handling a team of actors: '[m]y way of dealing with the stress of it was to say, well, I'm not going to be a director. I'm not going to tell people how to act, I'll tell them to freeze' (in Verhagen 2009: 3–4).

6 Her point is justified: 'I used the interview almost as a pool of words from which to edit new sentences and new thoughts that were not said in any interview' (Fast in Balsom, 2013: 151).

7 In this light, it is useful to recall an admittedly dubious experiment documented by Leys in which investigators found that 'viewers experienced presentations as pleasant when pictures and language coincided' (2017: 319). Their results led them to propose that this might also explain 'the well-documented finding that viewers recall TV news programs poorly, suggesting that the discrepancy between emotional pictures and the factual language employed in such programs interferes with comprehension and recall' (Leys, 2017: 319).

8 He is referring here to Brecht's Verfremdungseffekt or distanciation effect.

9 On the other hand, according to Ruth Leys, recent literature on transgenerational trauma by Caruth and others focuses on how the original foreclosed event of memory reappears intact and unrepresentable in the next generation. See her masterful *Trauma: A Genealogy* (2000).

10 By contrast to Laplanche's generative account of symbolization in relation to the enigmatic signifier, Ruth Leys describes how recent literature on transgenerational trauma by Caruth and others focuses on how the original

foreclosed event of memory reappears intact and unrepresentable in the next generation, a position that Leys critiques as unscientific.

11 Siqiao Lu, in an unpublished graduate essay, proposes that there is another public involved in the therapeutic aspect of this work, an inner public comprising the veterans themselves and their families that she refers to as a subaltern counter-public (https://nyu.academia.edu/SiqiaoLu, accessed 7 May 2018).

12 See https://vimeo.com/92063206, accessed 7 May 2018. On this panel, art historian Rosalyn Deutsche stated that art such as Wodiczko's works on the unconscious level whereby each viewer has to turn inwards to question themselves, which to my mind is a kind of liberal preaching to the converted.

13 Needless to say, this is a Western perspective and that trauma operates differently in a war zone in which there is a constant state of alert and imminent threat of being killed.

14 Harbord (2007) discusses this in relation to Michael Haneke's *Code Unknown* (2000).

15 A literary parallel for this form of acting out is referenced in Richard Grusin's discussion of Don DeLillo's *The Falling Man* (2007) in which, after 9/11, the protagonist takes up gambling, his interest or need being less the moment of the coup, but in the comfort that in the gap between one game ending and another beginning, there will always be another game. The reassurance of this structure enables a dissociative processing of traumatic experience. See *Premediation: Affect and Mediality after 9/11* (2010).

16 Prior to this sequence, the real ex-drone operator describes the difference between operating Predator, the drone surveillance technology, and playing computer games to unwind, as the camera's aerial view zooms into and then back from a scene of a rural idyllic US town. The free-floating aerial point-of-views of both sequences echo the operator's dissociation between the image of surveillance and the technology's capacity for killing. Drone operators often play computer games to unwind, as their first-person address give the illusion of being in control of one's target, whereas surveillance technology controls those who operate it. Describing research at MIT into monitoring the affective changes undergone by computer game players interactions, Grusin (2010) reports that the biggest increases in adrenaline occurred not when players were engaged in stressful, life-threatening battle, but when the software failed to work properly, thereby disrupting the feedback loop between player and game (111). Grusin proposes that the constancy of the low-level affective states produced by playing first-person shooter games may serve as a way for people to regulate anxiety,

keeping turbulence at a minimum (112). It is not a stretch of the imagination to apply this finding to why drone operators might find playing computer games relaxing.

17 Matt Delmont cites a 2012 report by International Human Rights and Conflict Resolution Clinic (Stanford Law School) and Global Justice Clinic (NYU School of Law), called 'Living under Drones', which asserts that constant drone surveillance and the persistent threat of missile strikes produce constant anxiety and psychological trauma for the Pakistani population. See Delmont (2013), 'Drone Encounters: Noor Behram, Omer Fast, and Visual Critiques of Drone Warfare', *American Quarterly*, 65 (1), p. 193.

18 See Susan Buck-Morss' 'Aesthetics and Anaesthetics: Walter Benjamin's Artwork Essay Reconsidered' (1992) for a compelling interpretation of Benjamin.

19 See the collection Annette Kuhn (ed.), *Little Madness: Winnicott, Transitional Phenomena and Cultural Experience* (London and New York: I.B. Tauris, 2013).

Chapter 5

1 Much of Berardi's analysis of semiotics and resistance is inspired by his encounter with Guattari.

2 Gilligan's following online series' *Popular Unrest* also has a gallery installation format. Phase 1 of *The Common Sense* was initially released online with the announcement that Phases 2A and 2B would follow, but, at the time of writing, the work is solely exhibited as a gallery installation.

3 The scenes were filmed at Pergola and Hill Garden, Hampstead Heath, London.

4 In Gilligan's subsequent three-episode video *Self-Capital* (2009), capitalism's sickness was mapped onto the body of the female actress who played all four roles in the film of Capital, Patient, Therapist and Receptionist. Using meditation and psychodynamic role-play to renew and revitalize the body of Capital, the video demonstrated how alternative therapies associated with 1960s and 1970s counterculture are co-opted by the entrepreneurial ethos of neoliberal cognitive capitalism as techniques to produce happy healthy workers, e.g. Wellness rooms in Apple and Google manufacturing sites.

5 For an account of capitalism and creative destruction, see Magagnoli (2013: 723–34).

6 As opposed to Stiegler's notion that the technological is the default condition of the human, Berardi hints at a phenomenological human experience outside

of the technological. However, for both of them, the connective flows of information that aggregate in cognitive capitalism short-circuit the durational longevity of relations over time.

7 Creative destruction, which for Schumpeter precipitated the end of capitalism as unsustainable, has been transformed by high-tech business demagogues into the trope of constant mutation and revolution in the development of new markets and new products such as Big Data. See William Davies, *The Limits of Neoliberalism: Authority, Sovereignty and the Logic of Competition* (Los Angeles, California: Sage, 2014), for more on Schumpeter's concept in relation to neoliberalism.

8 Gilligan explicitly states her goal is to change the world, her main motivation being a 'political commitment to changing the economic and political system we live in and striving toward another, better one' (in Donovan, 2012).

9 See Jean-Claude Polack's chapter 'Analysis, between Psycho and Schizo', in *The Guattari Effect* (eds.) Alliez and Goffey (Continuum, 2011), for an extensive account of Guattari's professional life at La Borde clinic and his political affiliations.

10 Interestingly, Gilligan also refers to the unconscious as the most powerful network processor known to man in her script for *Crisis in the Credit System*. See https://www.artangel.org.uk/project/crisis-in-the-credit-system/, accessed 7 November 2016. The performative imbrication of a-signifying semiotics and signifying semiologies is also manifest in Hito Steyerl's films, especially *Liquidity Inc.* (2014).

11 PayPal co-founder Peter Thiel is not only a supporter of the Trump administration thought to have manipulated data to get into power, but Palantir, the CIA-backed start-up he went on to found, operates Big Data analytics. I was alerted to this at a performance lecture 'Metric Mysticism' given by the artist Zach Blas at Edel Assanti gallery in London on 26 February 2019.

12 Although Lazzarato takes issue with the term in his essay Does Cognitive Capitalism Exist? (2014b), he nonetheless addresses it as a theory that attempts to capture the relationship between capitalism and processes of subjectivation in his earlier *Signs and Machines* (2014: 11).

13 This citation is from Gilligan's statement in the gallery press release when all fifteen episodes were shown at Edinburgh School of Fine Art during the Edinburgh Arts Festival 2018.

14 Although when Episode 1 of the work premiered online in May 2015 on Rhizomes.org, it was announced that the full series would be available soon after on www.thecommonsense.org.

15 While most are frontal, many of them are tilted, one or two towards the floor, which on my encounter with the work in Edinburgh led to a gallery visitor, who happened to be a clinical psychologist, sitting down on one of the screens thinking it was a seat. Needless to say, this real implosion resulted in the image becoming an a-semiotic glitch frozen on the surface as the monitor cracked.

Chapter 6

1 As Shaviro notes in *No Speed Limit*, while the term was first coined disparagingly by Noys in 2010, it has been repurposed as a positive term, most notably by Alex Williams and Nick Srnicek in their *Manifesto for an Accelerationist Politics* (2013), http://criticallegalthinking.com/2013/05/14/accelerate-manifesto-for-an-accelerationist-politics/, accessed 4 November 2019.

2 *I Feel Your Pain* was an eighty-minute live film performance commissioned by Performa 11 and held at the School of Visual Arts theatre in New York. Its fourteen vignettes were performed by eight actors from within the audience, while Laser acted as a real-time editor selecting which shots of the vignettes would appear on the screen in front of the audience. The work also involved three cinematographers and included a Chaplinesque silent clown and a disembodied announcer, both figures modelled on characters derived from 'The Living Newspaper', a type of theatre which emerged in the Soviet Union in the early 1920s and later migrated to the federal theatre projects of the Works Progress Administration funded by the US government.

3 Note that the script included editorial contributions from Scott Indrisek, Wendy Osserman, Jess Wilcox and Tom Williams.

4 https://www.youtube.com/watch?v=31Vr6F47fGc published on 29 June 2012, accessed 7 March 2017.

5 The work was a Performa 11 commission. When I first began researching it in 2017, one of the comments following the edited video iteration of this work on YouTube read: 'Propaganda only works on the converted, to everyone else it is just funny.' At the time of writing, this comment no longer exists online, though to my mind it neatly sums up the tendency for overt political art to speak to those who agree with its premise.

6 See Mannoni [1969] (2003: 68–92). Although my use of Mannoni's phrase is more of an aside, it is perhaps no coincidence that it has been used to discuss recent political events such as Brexit, the UK's withdrawal from the EU. See Burman (2018: 119–43).

7 Best and Sedgwick are here obliquely referencing Melanie Klein's psychoanalytic theories in which she splits the ego's developmental phases into two: the paranoid-schizoid and the depressive phase. While many readers view the latter phase in purely reparative terms, Sedgwick and Best rightly point out that the depressive phase not only has its own aggressivity, but that the relation between the two phases is not linear.

8 To coincide with the installation, Laser also holds public events called Political Therapy workshops. Members of the public register to attend these, the price being similar to an exhibition entrance ticket. Performance works in their own right, they are hosted by a therapist or life coach to address political crises that are relevant to the workshops' location. For example, the press release for a workshop held at the performance festival Block Universe in London in 2017 stated that 'Laser has enlisted drama therapist and actress Louise Platt to guide participants through activities that facilitate the expression of frustrations related to Brexit and other current events', http://blockuniverse.co.uk/political-therapy-workshop/, accessed 2 June 2017. Workshops have taken place in advance of the 2016 presidential election at Brooklyn Academy of Music, New York; in the UK before Article 50 was initiated at Grand Union, Birmingham; at CAC Brétigny between the first and second rounds of France's presidential elections; and at Jupiter Artland Foundation, near Edinburgh, where participants addressed the debates surrounding Scottish independence.

9 My encounter with the installation was at CAC Brétigny in 2017. There, the therapist was played by Adele Jacques, her direct-to-camera address and mellifluous voice immediately working on me, as I sat on the grey mattress and lay back on one of the pillows in an echo of the actors lying on similar pillows on-screen.

10 See James Nolan's *The Therapeutic State: Justifying Government at Century's End* (1998) for an account of therapeutic governance in the US.

11 Jane Bradley, in *The Scotsman*, 24 March 2017, cites John Heffernan, head of exhibitions at Jupiter Artland, Scotland, describing a political therapy workshop he took part in at an art gallery in Birmingham: 'I think, like many people, I rarely talk to people who have different political opinions to me. I discuss issues with my friends over dinner, but we generally have the same beliefs. The course coaches you through doing that without being hateful and aggressive.

When you sit down, you initially do not reveal what your political opinions are. It was only during the workshop that you got an intuition as to what people thought, but by that time, you have been brought to the way of thinking that it is OK to disagree about politics.' https://www.pressreader.com/uk/the-scotsman/20170324/281788513886610, accessed 31 January 2020. Although his view is bound to be positive, given that Jupiter Artland exhibited *Primal Speech* in 2017, it nonetheless highlights the potential solidarity of those who have nothing in common.

12 Lauren Berlant (2011) suggests that this flourishing might not be necessarily aspirational but more a kind of hanging out in creative ways in a present full of obstacles.

13 Initially presented as a paper to the New York Psychoanalytic Society in 1968, the chapter 'The Use of an Object and Relating through Identifications' is included in Winnicott's *Playing and Reality* ([1971] 2001).

Chapter 7

1 Here my use of 'actants' refers to Bruno Latour's actor-network theory which maintains that all the interrelating entities in an environment comprise its actants or actors. This includes both human and non-human actors. See Latour's *Reassembling the Social: An Introduction to Actor-Network Theory* (Oxford and New York: Oxford University Press, 2005).

2 The Tavistock Institute of Human Relations (TIHR) applies social science to contemporary issues and problems. It was established as a not-for-profit organization with charitable purpose in 1947. https://www.tavinstitute.org/who-we-are/, accessed 27 February 2020.

3 For a history of Spence's therapeutic photography prior to her work with Martin, see Terry Dennett's 'Jo Spence's Camera Therapy: Personal Therapeutic Photography as a Response to Adversity', *European Journal of Psychotherapy & Counselling*, 11 (1) (2009), pp.7–19.

4 Spence later enacted photo therapy work with other collaborators such as her partner David Roberts. Prior to her photo therapy work with Martin, she had collaborated with her then-partner Terry Dennett on projects such as *Remodelling Photo History (The History Lesson)* (1982).

5 Admittedly, the dialogic nature of this collaboration is somewhat foreclosed by exhibitions that present this work as static photographs. For example, while Martin is credited as a collaborator, her side of the work as 'creative director' is rarely, if ever, shown. Terry Dennett describes their process: 'the sitter becomes creative director while the photographer's role is elevated to that of therapist; the camera operation is then seen as a simple technical process. After each session

the roles are reversed, and the previous photographer becomes the new creative director. Each then has full creative management of their own sessions and ownership of their session films afterwards' (2009: 15).

6 The programme was adapted from Project STEEP (Steps toward Effective Enjoyable Parenting), an intervention developed in the United States in response to 'The Parent Child Project', a study implemented in 1975 by Egeland, Deinard and Stroufe.

7 See Benjamin's 'The Work of Art in the Age of Mechanical Reproduction' [1935] in *Illuminations: Essays and Reflections*, ed. and trans. Hannah Arendt (London: Jonathan Cape, 1970), pp.166–95. Benjamin states, 'The camera introduces us to unconscious optics as does psychoanalysis to unconscious impulses' (189).

8 At the time of writing, it is available to view on the artists' website at https://leighledare.com/Zurich-Large-Group, accessed 4 March 2020.

9 The Tavistock Method is essentially: (a) a method of analysis of institutions, aiming at action-research or organizational diagnosis; (b) a training tool for managers, technicians and professionals; (c) a consultancy technique for organizations that are going through some difficulty and their members. For further information, see https://www.ilnodogroup.it/en/areas-of-activity/work-method/tavistock-method, accessed 31 May 2019.

10 My notes from the post-screening Q&A at https://ly.yes-vlip.lv/video/%2FPYcsYQAXHEy%2Bmo%3D.html, accessed 17 March 2019.

11 A group relations conference is a personal development programme, which aims to increase your personal effectiveness in any organizational role. Development happens through experiential learning – you will learn from the immediate experience of participation in, and reflection on, the conference event. https://tavistockandportman.nhs.uk/news-and-events/group-relations-conferences/, accessed 17 June 2019

12 Email to author, 11 July 2019.

13 Ibid.

14 See the post-screening Q&A with Ledare at the 2018 Sheffield documentary film festival at https://ly.yes-vlip.lv/video/%2FPYcsYQAXHEy%2Bmo%3D.html, accessed 17 March 2019.

15 See the artist's website: https://leighledare.com/The-Task, accessed 17 June 2019.

16 Guattari also posits that even at the a-semiotic level of signification, which I referred to in Chapter 3, the message transmitted to the child from the pregnant woman 'concerns industrial society' (Guattari, 2015: 84).

17 In response to interviewer Oliver Zahm's provocation that contemporary artists' work often comprises discursive narrative and fiction, Guattari asserts

that 'the subjective mutation made by aesthetic refrain is not discursive, it is the outbreak of the non-discursive at the heart of the discursive' (in Guattari and Zahm, 2011: 47). By contrast to my appropriation of his writings on cinema as offering a mode of resistance to dominant signification, Guattari maintains that it is only painting that has the capacity to create 'mutant percepts and affects' that resist the 'homogenesis of capitalism' (in Guattari and Zahm, 2011: 42–4).

Chapter 8

1 A few years after writing this, I read a review of Stiegler's *What Makes Life Worth Living* in which the authors claim that 'the relationship between rigidity and tolerance in psychoanalysis helps us to delineate the pharmakon as a *relational remedy*' (Voela and Rothschild, 2019: 58, my emphasis).

2 The initial performance of the show was live streamed on www.stickam.com. This is no longer available.

3 Parker and Sedgwick say: 'Where Austin, then, seemed intent on separating the actor's citational practices from ordinary speech-act performances, Derrida regarded both as structured by a generalized iterability, a pervasive theatricality common to stage and world alike' (1995: 4).

4 See Furedi (2004), pp.84–105.

5 My notes based on a conversation with the artist in London on 8 July 2019. She underscores this notion in her unpublished PhD thesis, describing her practice as 'a methodology that is capable of challenging neoliberal values and norms in utilising what might be deemed its very own inward-looking practices' (2019: 181).

6 I will have cause to return to this idea in the next chapter in relation to Michel Feher's essay 'Self-Appreciation: Or, The Aspirations of Human Capital', *Public Culture*, 21 (1) (2009).

7 Fox's mother, Angela Monti Fox, a psychodynamic psychoanalyst, is brought on as a guest in Episode 2 of *The O Show* to advise a performance artist friend of Fox's on her love life. Interestingly, Fox's father is a child psychologist.

8 Lean-in feminism is named as such after the book *Lean In: Women, Work, and the Will to Lead* (2013) by CEO of Facebook Sheryl Sandberg which advises women on how to succeed in the corporate world without sacrificing family life.

9 Fox, 'Introducing the O Show', Performance Matters, 30 May 2012, http://www.thisisperformancematters.co.uk/potentials-of-performance/words-and-images.post125.html, accessed 6 January 2016.

10 Cited from Episode 3, Part 4 https://www.youtube.com/watch?v=sq21e4dy_Kk, accessed 6 January 2016.

11 Email correspondence between the author and Fox, 27 October 2016.

12 In using the term 'truth-effect' I am loosely combining Michel Foucault's notion of a 'regime of truth' with J.L. Austin's notion of how both felicitous and infelicitous performatives prompt actions. For Austin, performative statements are neither true nor false but happy (felicitous) or unhappy (infelicitous). An infelicitous (unhappy) performative might not deliver on an act, for example, of promising something to someone, but nonetheless the utterance produces a 'truth-effect' in prompting another's response. Foucault's regime of truth is also performative. It describes: 'the types of discourse which [each society] accepts and makes function as true; the mechanisms and instances which enable one to distinguish true and false statements, the means by which each is sanctioned; *the techniques and procedures accorded value in the acquisition of truth*; the status of those who are charged with saying what counts as true' (Foucault in Rabinow, 1984, p.73, my emphasis).

13 Hirsch, 'gURLS Performance Text', n.d., http://therealannhirsch.com/misc.html, accessed 17 December 2014. In an email correspondence between Fox and the author, Fox notes the common ground between her work and Hirsch's in this respect.

14 For more information on Hirsch in relation to performative subjectivities and resistance, see my essay 'Performing Resistance to Performing Autonomy and Back Again: Alex Bag Meets Ann Hirsch' in *MIRAJ: Moving Image Review and Art Journal*, 4(1 & 2) (2015), pp.13–41.

15 Interestingly, Kurtz puts forward a more relational approach to projection, claiming that 'we project into others those part of ourselves which we want to get rid of, or not know about […] that we actively, if unconsciously, invite others to know something about us that we do not know about ourselves' (in Coetzee and Kurtz, 2015: 140).

16 For a different approach to the transformative potential of performance, see Fischer-Lichte (2008).

17 Sergei Prozorov, 'Foucault's Affirmative Biopolitics: Cynic Parrhesia and the Biopower of the Powerless', *Political Theory*, 45 (6) (2017), pp.801–23. Article first published online: 9 October 2015, https://journals.sagepub.com/doi/abs/10.1177/0090591715609963, accessed 7 October 2019.

18 Email correspondence between the author and Fox, 27 October 2016.

19 Ibid.

20 See Oriana Fox's 'Performance Art Can Change Your Life! Shame Attacking and *Parrhesia* as Feminist Practices of Freedom', PhD thesis, London: Goldsmiths University (2018), especially pp.24–9.

21 These lectures were developed subsequent to Foucault's diagnosis of neoliberal entrepreneurialism in *The Birth of Biopolitics* (1978).

22 A recent art example of enclosed small groups for the purposes of pedagogical medicinal care is Simone Leigh's *The Waiting Room* (2016), presented at the New Museum, New York in 2016. Describing the relatively empty gallery room, curator Helen Molesworth suggests that 'the real work lay elsewhere, namely, in the workshops on such topics as complementary medicine, folk-healing traditions, acupuncture, and meditation. Many of these events occurred while the museum was closed to the public, notably *Home Economics*, a program designed specifically for fifteen black schoolgirls, investigating ways to address the holistic needs of black women in relation to wellness and the medical establishment' (2018). While socially engaged practice is beyond the remit of my book, Molesworth makes a good case for such practices of self-care in a political context in which young black women are doubly discriminated against by being both hypervisible and invisible.

23 Subsequent to publishing an earlier version of this chapter in 2017, https://necsus-ejms.org/acts-of-laughter-acts-of-tears-the-production-of-truth-effects-in-oriana-foxs-the-o-show-and-gillian-wearings-self-made/, I discovered that Fox was actually inspired by Wearing's work.

24 http://selfmade.org.uk/gillian/, accessed 2 June 2017.

25 In one of the ten instalments, Wearing, her back facing the viewer, appears to the side of the screen like a faux therapist. In the 1990s and 2000s, this work was received as a critique of reality TV, as was Phil Collin's more overtly deconstructionist four-channel video installation *gerçeğin geri dönüşü* [*the return of the real*] (2005), in which four micro-celebrities of Turkish reality TV describe how participating in such shows had impacted their lives in often negative ways. More recently, film historian Catherine Fowler reframes both Wearing's and Collins's works in relation to 'the contemporary proliferation of recordings of ordinary people performing on reality television and on the Internet' (2013: 11). This new context is more about their emotional resonance than critique.

26 The other two participants' 'end films' are included the DVD extras.

27 It is interesting to note that when Boal later worked in Europe in the mid-1970s, he had to adapt *Theatre of the Oppressed* to address 'oppressions' of a more 'psychological, esoteric, and metaphysical' kind such as feelings of loneliness

and emptiness as opposed to the social and political oppressions such as police brutality and unemployment that had characterized his political activism in Brazil and Argentina. However, as Mady Schutzman states, his techniques 'have always interfaced with therapeutic ones [...] his "spect-actor" scheme relevant to *all* social transformations' (1994: 137).

28 Although, according to Boal, Aristotle referred to catharsis only once in his text on tragedy, *Poetics*, it has nonetheless become synonymous with Aristotelian theatre. See Boal (2008: 23).

29 For more on Brecht's theories of theatre, see Brecht (1974).

30 Recall here Winnicott's 'Fear of Breakdown' that I discussed in Chapter 6.

31 See Philip Auslander's *From Acting to Performance: Essays in Modernism and Postmodernism* (London and New York: Routledge, 1999), p.99.

32 'What is realised in my history is not the past definite of what was, since it is no more, or even the present perfect of what has been in what I am, but the future anterior of what I shall have been for what I am in the process of becoming' (Lacan [1966] 1977: 86).

Chapter 9

1 This is a screen title from Maria Ruido's video *Real Time* (2003) which is quoted in Amy Charlesworth, 'Caught between the Factory and the Home', *Third Text*, 29 (1–2) (2015), pp. 88–103, p.89.

2 Federici was one of the group of women who founded the International Wages For Housework Campaign in Italy in 1972, which was linked to Italian workerism or *operaismo*, proponents of which include Negri and Berardi. Federici went on to found Wages for Housework in 1973 in New York. It is worth noting that this campaign influenced film collective projects in Britain such as *Women of the Rhondda* (dir. Mary Capps and Mary Kelly, 1973) and The Berwick Street Film Collective's *Nightcleaners* (1972–75). See Hana Janečková's web project online at http://artycok.tv/en/26980/novy-feminismus-nektere-zeny-jine-zeny-a-vsichni-ti-zahorkli-pivarinew-feminism-some-women-other-women-and-all-the-bittermen (accessed 21 October 2015) for a connection between Zaman's film and the campaign. Note too that for Federici, the campaign for reproductive labour to be salaried was not simply to put housework on a par with male industrial labour but part of a move to 'reorganise it as creative' (in Vishmidt, 2013).

3 Beech sees these two short films as companion pieces both being 'fictional workshops in "emotion entrepreneurship"', email correspondence with author, 29 February 2016.
4 *The Pain of Others* (dir. Penny Lane, 2018), a found footage documentary film about women who suffer from Morgellons, communicates how this disease is both exacerbated and alleviated by online sharing.
5 This citation is from Beech's notes on the film sent to the author in an email correspondence, 29 February 2016.
6 In relation to *Pharmakon*, Beech contrasts the notion of well-being to the biomedical model which she views as a way of 'seeing disease', or of 'seeing the body' that is often constructed from a very narrow view (very often male). Email correspondence with the author, 29 February 2016.
7 Note that this is not dissimilar to my exploration of both Method and Boalian theatre in the previous chapter.
8 The phrase 'comic crownings and uncrownings' in particular.
9 The work drew on the cultural metaphor of Oswald de Andrade in his 'Manifesto Antropofago' (1928) which claimed that Brazilian artists needed to cannibalize the Western other and excrete it, so to speak, to gain credence in the global art world. The metaphor of cannibalism is borrowed from anthropology, but it also links to psychoanalysis and the cannibalistic incorporation of the other in the construction of identity in the early phases of development.
10 *Some Women, Other Women and All the Bittermen* was commissioned by The Tetley in Leeds and was the outcome of Zaman's residency there which involved a twelve-month process of doing research in The Tetley archive, interviewing ex-Tetley's Brewery workers, as well as co-running workshops with women from the recently formed Leeds branch of *Justice for Domestic Workers* (J4DW). The workshops were supported by curator and writer Amy Charlesworth, J4DW (London), Gill Park, Director of visual arts organization Pavilion, and artists Jo Dunn and Terry Wragg from Leeds Animation Workshop.
11 Aside from unregulated work conditions, Domestic Workers are subject to the UK government's rescinding of their visa rights in 2012, making it impossible for them to change employer. This is the key issue that is discussed in the workshops in Zaman's film.
12 For more on this shift, see Charlotte Brunsdon's 'Crossroads: Notes on Soap Opera', *Screen*, 22 (4) (1981), pp.32–7; and, more recently, Rosalind Gill's 'Culture and subjectivity in neoliberal and postfeminist times', *Subjectivity*, 25 (2008), pp.432–45.

13 Zaman's video can be seen in the context of the historical reception of The Berwick Street Film Collective's *Nightcleaners*, 1972–1975, a documentary film about the campaign led by activist and night cleaner May Hobbs to set up a grassroots organization to unionize the immigrant and working-class women who performed this invisible labour. Many feminists and activists criticized *Nightcleaners* for its aesthetic formalism. For an account of this, see Wilson (2015), pp.25–7. See also Sheila Rowbotham, 'Jolting Memory: *Nightcleaners* Recalled', in Maria Ruido (ed.), *Plan Rosebud: On Images, Sites and Politics of Memory* (CGAC, Santiago de Compostela, 2008), p.13. Thanks to Rehana Zaman for sending me Rowbotham's text.

14 See Gayatri Chakravorty Spivak's 'Can the Subaltern Speak' (1988) in which she critiques Foucault's and Deleuze's and Guattari's liberal aesthetics in this light.

15 Terry Wragg and Jo Dunn from the Leeds Animation Workshop later made an animation campaign film in consultation with the domestic workers titled *They Call Us Maids: The Domestic Workers' Story* (2015).

16 In this essay, Feher's only example of turning neoliberalism's imperative of self-reliance from something exploitative into something collectively productive is the Scandinavian labour unions who, rather than rejecting workfare programmes, work through them by deploying a concept of 'flexsecurity'.

17 This panel was part of the curatorial programme 'Now You Can Go' which was developed by participants from the Feminist Duration Reading Group coordinated by Helena Reckitt with Dimitra Gkitsa and including Angelica Bollettenari, Giulia Casalini, Diana Georgiou, Laura Guy, Irene Revell and Amy Tobin.

Chapter 10

1 Referring to examples such as Oscar Wilde, glam rock and Michel Foucault's care of the self, Shaviro admits that aesthetic self-cultivation has historically acted as a secret secession from dominant power rather than a resistance within it.

2 For a critique of this mode of aesthetic cultivation and privilege in relation to Miranda July's films, see D'Ambrose (2011). Interestingly, July is also referred to by Berardi (2011: 42) as one of two contemporary artists, the other being Eija-Liisa Ahtila, whose work exemplifies the neuro-psychopathologies of semiocapitalism.

3 Here one could think of the work of artist Carolyn Lazard and the popularity in artistic circles of Johanna Hedva's 'Sick Woman Theory' (http://www.maskmagazine.com/not-again/struggle/sick-woman-theory, accessed 22

March 2018). Thanks to Ilona Sagar for initially alerting me to this text. For an introduction to Lazard's work in the context of self-care, see Giulia Smith's profile of the artist in *Art Monthly*, 429 (September 2019), pp.15–16.

4 As Larne Abse Gogarty cogently puts it in her critique of this instrumentalization in ' "Usefulness" in Contemporary Art and Politics': 'When contemporary artists attempt to reanimate individuals and communities who have otherwise been condemned as disposable [...] this all too often involves, in the present, taking on aspects of social reproduction to "repurpose" those populations and make them "useful" along lines that draw tacit support from the state and capital' (*Third Text*, 31 (1) (2017), pp.117–32, p.131).

5 Admittedly, the partial abstraction of my pharmacological framework pales before the activist context of Lorde's notion of '[v]isualizing the disease process inside my body in political images' (1988: 132).

6 In his article '*Mad Men* and Mindfulness', Niels Niessen critiques 'practices of mindfulness meditation for their ideology of a centered, *lovingkind* individual whose attention remains unperturbed by the economic seasons' (2018: 275, original emphasis). However, he also makes what to my mind is a pharmacological argument that the equation of attention and everyday life in mindfulness discourses can also be used to redraw boundaries between work and leisure, thereby providing protection from the colonization of the mind in cognitive capitalism. See *Discourse*, 40(3), (Fall 2018), pp. 273–307.

7 Kisner further critiques #selfcare as follows: 'The irony of the grand online #selfcare-as-politics movement of 2016 is that it was powered by straight, affluent white women, who, although apparently feeling a new vulnerability in the wake of the election, are not traditionally the segment of American society in the greatest need of affirmation' (https://www.newyorker.com/culture/culture-desk/the-politics-of-selfcare, accessed 1 October 2017).

8 While I have seen *Toxic* in different iterations at the South London Gallery, London in 2013 and at Ellen de Bruijne Projects, Amsterdam in 2012, I refer to it here less as one of my particular case studies, but more as a theoretical reference in Engel's and Lorenz's article which allows me to expand on the toxic pole of the pharmacological.

9 Hamja Ashan made a similar point in his guest appearance on *The O Show* in Chapter 8.

10 Coincidently, I was in the audience and can verify the intensity of this discussion. Zaman also makes reference to feminist filmmaker Michelle Citron's *What You Take for Granted* (1983–1984). Strand's experimental documentary presents five

female friends who speak direct-to-camera about their sexuality and ambivalent desires, blending these talking head portraits with sequences of lyrical abstraction.

11 Thanks to artist Ima-Abasi Okon for re-alerting me to this context.

12 Zaman characterizes the beauty salon as 'a space where inter-corporeality and pleasure is offered as an alternative to the anxieties of collective experience' https://lux.org.uk/work/025217-sharla-shabana-sojourner-selena, accessed 6 December 2017.

13 As Jessica Benjamin argues in relation to the mother–child interrelation, asymmetry does not necessarily exclude the mutuality of pleasure and autonomy. See Benjamin (2018).

14 See Walsh (2016).

15 Here I am referring back to my earlier discussion of Walter Benjamin's narcotic insulation/inoculation.

Bibliography

Ahmed, S., 2004. *The Cultural Politics of Emotion*. Edinburgh: Edinburgh University Press.

Alexander, S., 2016. D.W. Winnicott and the Social Democratic Vision. In: M. ffytche and D. Pick, eds. *Psychoanalysis in the Age of Totalitarianism*. Abingdon and New York: Routledge.

Archey, K., 2012. *Artist Profile: Ann Hirsch*. [online] Rhizome. Available at: http://rhizome.org/editorial/2012/mar/7/artist-profile/ [Accessed 19 October. 2015].

Auslander, P., 1999. *From Acting to Performance: Essays in Modernism and Postmodernism*. London and New York: Routledge.

Austin, J.L., Sbisá, M. and Urmson, J.O., 1976. *How to Do Things with Words*. 2nd ed. William James lectures. Oxford: Oxford University Press.

Bainbridge, C., Ward, I. and Yates, C. eds., 2014. *Television and Psychoanalysis: Psycho-cultural Perspectives*. London: Karnac Books.

Balsom, E., 2013. *Exhibiting Cinema in Contemporary Art*. Amsterdam, Netherlands: Amsterdam: University Press.

Beech, D., 2017. Projecting the Future: Krzysztof Wodiczko Interviewed by Dave Beech. *Art Monthly*, (409), September, pp.1–4.

Beller, J., 2006. *The Cinematic Mode of Production: Attention Economy and the Society of the Spectacle*. Hanover, NH, London: University Press of New England.

Benjamin, J., 2018. *Beyond Doer and Done To: Recognition Theory, Intersubjectivity and the Third*. London and New York: Routledge.

Bennett, J., 2005. *Empathic Vision: Affect, Trauma, and Contemporary Art*. Stanford, CA: Stanford University Press.

Bennett, J., 2012. *Practical Aesthetics: Events, Affect and Art after 9/11*. London: I.B. Tauris.

Berardi, F.B., 2007. Sensitivity to the Rhizome. *16 Beaver*. [online] Available at: http://16beavergroup.org/journalisms/2007/02/13/franco-berardi-bifo-sensitivity-to-the-rhizome/ [Accessed 6 June 2018].

Berardi, F.B., 2009. *The Soul at Work: From Alienation to Autonomy*. Translated by F. Cadel G. Mecchia. Los Angeles, CA: Semiotext(e).

Berardi, F.B., 2010. Cognitarian Subjectivation. *e-flux*, [online] 20, November. Available at: https://www.e-flux.com/journal/20/67633/cognitarian-subjectivation/ [Accessed 6 June 2018].

Berardi, F.B., 2011. *After the Future*. Translated by A. Bove. Oakland, CA, Edinburgh: AK Press.

Berardi, F.B., 2012. *Emancipation of the Sign: Poetry and Finance during the Twentieth Century. e-flux*, [online] (39). Available at: https://www.e-flux.com/journal/39/60284/emancipation-of-the-sign-poetry-and-finance-during-the-twentieth-century/ [Accessed 22 October 2019].

Berardi, F.B., 2013. The Mind's We: Morphogenesis and the Chaosmic Spasm. In: W. Neidich and A. De Boever, eds. *The Psychopathologies of Cognitive Capitalism, Part One*. Berlin: Archive Books. pp.7–32.

Berardi, F.B., 2014. *And. Phenomenology of the End. Cognition and Sensibility in the Transition from Conjunctive to Connective Mode of Social Communication*. Aalto: Aalto ARTS Books.

Berardi, F.B., 2017. *Futurability: The Age of Impotence and the Horizon of Possibility.* London and New York: Verso Books.

Berlant, L.G., 2011. *Cruel Optimism*. Durham: Duke University Press.

Berlant, L.G. and Povinelli, E.A., 2014. Holding Up the World, Part III: In the Event of Precarity'. A Conversation. *e-flux*, [online] (58), October. Available at: https://www.e-flux.com/journal/58/61149/holding-up-the-world-part-iii-in-the-event-of-precarity-a-conversation/ [Accessed 1 October 2019].

Bernes, J.J., 2015. Capital and Community: On Melanie Gilligan's Trilogy. *Mute*. Available at: https://www.metamute.org/editorial/articles/capital-and-community-melanie-gilligan%E2%80%99s-trilogy [Accessed 7 June 2017].

Bersani, L., 1990. *The Culture of Redemption*. Cambridge, MA: Harvard University Press.

Best, S., 2016. *Reparative Aesthetics; Witnessing in Contemporary Art Photography*. London and New York: Bloomsbury.

Bion, W.R., 1961. *Experiences in Groups and other Papers*. 2004th ed. London and New York: Taylor & Francis e-Library.

Bion, W.R., 1990. *Brazilian Lectures: 1973, Sao Paulo; 1974, Rio de Janeiro/Sao Paulo*. London: Karnac Books.

Biressi, A. and Nunn, H., 2005. *Reality TV: Realism and Revelation*. London: Wallflower.

Bishop, C., 2004. Antagonism and Relational Aesthetics. *October*, (110), pp.51–79.

Bishop, C., 2012. Delegated Performance: Outsourcing Authenticity. *October*, 140, pp.91–112.

Boal, A., 1995. *The Rainbow of Desire: The Boal Method of Theatre and Therapy*. Translated by A. Jackson. London, New York: Routledge.

Boal, A., 2008. *Theatre of the Oppressed*. 3rd ed. Translated by C.A. and M.-O. Leal McBride. London, England: Pluto.

de Botton, A. and Armstrong, J., 2016. *Art as Therapy*. London: Phaidon Press.

Bourriaud, N., 2002. *Relational Aesthetics*. Documents sur l'art. Translated by S. Pleasance and F. Woods. Paris: Les presses du réel.

Brady, S., 2012. *Performance, Politics, and the War on Terror: 'Whatever It Takes'*. Basingstoke: Palgrave Macmillan.

Brady, S., 2015. God, the Pilot, and the Bugsplat: Performance and the Drone Effect. *Behemoth: A Journal on Civilisation*, 8(2), pp.34–54.

Brady, S., 2016. The Soldier Cycle: Harun Farocki's Images of War (at a Distance). In: H. Bial and S. Brady, eds. *The Performance Studies Reader*, 3rd ed. Abingdon and New York: Routledge. pp.193–202.

Brandt, M.R., 2013. *War, Trauma, and Technologies of the Self: The Making of Virtual Reality Exposure Therapy*. [PhD] University of California San Diego. Available at: https://escholarship.org/content/qt6698t67t/qt6698t67t.pdf [Accessed 3 August 2019].

Brecht, B., 1974. *Brecht on Theatre: The Development of an Aesthetic*. Translated by J. Willett. London: Eyre Methuen.

Brenez, N., 2010. Harun Farocki and the Romantic Genesis of the Principle of Visual Critique. In: A. Ehmann and K. Eshun, eds. *Harun Farocki: Against What? Against Whom?* London: Koenig Books. pp.128–42.

Brunsdon, C., 1981. Crossroads: Notes on Soap Opera. *Screen*, 8(2), December, pp.32–7.

Buck-Morss, S., 1992. Aesthetics and Anaesthetics: Walter Benjamin's Artwork Essay Reconsidered. *October*, 62, pp.3–41.

Burman, E., 2018. Brexit, "Child as Method," and the Pedagogy of Failure: How Discourses of Childhood Structure the Resistance of Racist Discourse to Analysis. *Review of Education, Pedagogy, and Cultural Studies*, 40 (2), pp.119–43.

Butler, J., 1990. *Gender Trouble: Feminism and the Subversion of Identity*. London and New York: Routledge.

Butler, J., 1993. *Bodies That Matter: On the Discursive Limits of 'Sex'*. London and New York: Routledge.

Butler, J., 1997. *Excitable Speech: A Politics of the Performative*. New York and London: Routledge.

Campt, T.M., 2017. *Listening to Images*. Durham: Duke University Press.

Caruth, C., 1995. *Trauma: Explorations in Memory*. Baltimore, MD, London: Johns Hopkins University Press.

Caruth, C., 1996. *Unclaimed Experience: Trauma, Narrative, and History*. Baltimore, MD, London: Johns Hopkins University Press.

Celis Bueno, C., 2016. Reterritorialisation and Antiproduction in Harun Farocki's 'Eye/Machine' Trilogy. *Westminster Advanced Studies*, (3), pp.3–23.

Celis Bueno, C., 2017. *The Attention Economy: Labour, Time and Power in Cognitive Capitalism*. London and New York: Rowman and Littlefield.

Chamarette, J., 2015. The 'New' Experimentalism: Women In/And/On Film. In: L. Mulvey and A. Backman Rogers, eds. *Feminisms: Diversity, Difference and Multiplicity in Contemporary Film Cultures*. Amsterdam: Amsterdam University Press. pp.125–40.

Charlesworth, A., 2015. Caught between the Factory and the Home. *Third Text*, 29(1–2), pp.88–103.

Chinen, L., 2014. *At Our Expense: Harun Farocki's Images at War*. [online] Rhizome. Available at: https://rhizome.org/editorial/2014/jul/25/harun-farocki/ [Accessed 19 May 2018].

Coetzee, J.M. and Kurtz, A., 2015. *The Good Story: Exchanges on Truth, Fiction and Psychoanalytic Psychotherapy*. London: Harvill Secker.

D'Ambrose, R., 2011. The Aesthetic and the Therapeutic. *The Brooklyn Rail*. [online] December. Available at: https://brooklynrail.org/2011/12/film/the-aesthetic-and-the-therapeutic [Accessed 15 December 2017].

Davies, W., 2014. *The Limits of Neoliberalism: Authority, Sovereignty and the Logic of Competition*. Los Angeles, CA: Sage.

Davies, W., 2015. *The Happiness Industry: How the Government and Big Business Sold Us Well-Being*. London, England: Verso.

De Bruyn, D., 2014. *The Performance of Trauma in Moving Image Art*. Newcastle upon Tyne. Cambridge Scholars Publishing.

Deamer, D., 2012. Now You See Me … Gillian Wearing's 'Self Made'. In: D. Globus, D. Hermann and D. Krystof, eds. *Gillian Wearing*. London and Düsseldorf: Whitechapel Gallery/Ridinghouse/Kunstsammlung Nordhein-Westfalen. pp.39–45.

Dean, J., 2009. *Democracy and Other Neoliberal Fantasies: Communicative Capitalism and Left Politics*. Durham: Duke University Press.

Deleuze, Gilles and Guattari, Félix, 2000. *Anti-Oedipus: Capitalism and Schizophrenia*. R. Hurley, M. Seem & H.R. Lane Continuum.

Delmont, M., 2013. Drone Encounters: Noor Behram, Omer Fast, and Visual Critiques of Drone Warfare. *American Quarterly*, 65(1), pp.193–202.

Demos, T.J., 2012. War Games: A Tale in Three Parts. In: Milena Hoegsberg and Melanie O'Brian, eds. *Omer Fast: 5,000 Feet is the Best*. Berlin: Sternberg Press. pp.77–87.

Dennett, T., 2009. Jo Spence's Camera Therapy: Personal Therapeutic Photography as a Response to Adversity. *European Journal of Psychotherapy & Counselling*, 11(1), pp.7–19.

Derrida, J., 1981. Plato's Pharmacy. Translated by B. Johnson. In: *Dissemination*. Chicago: University of Chicago Press. pp.63–171.

Derrida, J., [1972] (1988). Signature Event Context. In: Samuel Weber and Jeffrey Mehlman, trans.. *Limited Inc.* Evanston, Il: Northwestern University Press.

Dolphijn, R. and van der Tuin, I., 2012. Interview with Rosi Braidotti. *New Materialism: Interviews & Cartographies.* [online] Open Humanities Press. pp.19–37. Available at: https://quod.lib.umich.edu/o/ohp/11515701.0001.001/1:4.1/--new-materialism-interviews-cartographies?rgn=div2;view=fulltext [Accessed 5 June 2016].

Donovan, T., 2012. *5 Questions for Contemporary Practice: Melanie Gilligan.* [online] Art21. Available at: http://magazine.art21.org/2012/05/22/5-questions-for-contemporary-practice-melanie-gilligan/#.XYzrdCWLmV4 [Accessed 4 November 2017].

Ecclestone, K. and Hayes, D., 2009. *The Dangerous Rise of Therapeutic Education.* London: Routledge.

Ehmann, A. and Eshun, K. eds., 2009. *Harun Farocki: Against What? Against Whom?* London: Koenig Books.

Ehmann, A. and Guerra, C. eds., 2016. *Harun Farocki: Another Kind of Empathy.* [online] London: Koenig Books. Available at: https://filmskemutacije.com/ANTJE-EHMANN-CARLES-GUERRA-HARUN-FAROCKI-DRUGA-VRSTA-EMPATIJE [Accessed 3 May 2015].

Engel, A. and Lorenz, R., 2013. Toxic Assemblages, Queer Socialities: A Dialogue of Mutual Poisoning. *e-flux*, [online] (44). Available at: <https://www.e-flux.com/journal/44/60173/toxic-assemblages-queer-socialities-a-dialogue-of-mutual-poisoning/> [Accessed 3 March 2014].

Eshun, K., 2012. Anaesthetising the Image: Immersion, Harun Farocki. In: J. Ten Brink and J. Oppenheimer, eds. *Killer Images: Documentary Film, Memory, and the Performance of Violence.* New York and Chicester West Sussex: Columbia University Press. pp.67–79.

Esposito, R., 2013. Community, Immunity, Biopolitics. Translated by Z. Hanafi. *Angelaki: Journal of the Theoretical Humanities*, 18(3), pp.83–90.

FACT, n.d. *FF Gaiden: Control.* [online] FACT. Available at: https://www.fact.co.uk/artwork/ff-gaiden-control [Accessed 19 August 2019].

FACETS, n.d. [online] Available at: https://www.facetsdvd.com/How-to-Live-in-the-German-Federal-Republic-p/dv99736.htm [Accessed 6 June 2017].

Farocki, H., 2009. How to Live in the FRG. In: A. Ehmann and K. Eshun, eds. *Harun Farocki: Against What? Against Whom?* London: Koenig Books. pp.163–5.

Farocki, H., 2012. Immersion (2009). In: J. Ten Brink and J. Oppenheimer, eds. *Killer Images: Documentary Film, Memory, and the Performance of Violence.* New York and Chicester West Sussex: Columbia University Press. pp.63–6.

Farocki, H., 2016. Einfühlung Empathy (2008). In: A. Ehmann and C. Guerra, eds. *Harun Farocki: Another Kind of Empathy*. London: Koenig Books. pp.104–5.

Federici, S., 2006. Precarious Labor: A Feminist Viewpoint. Available at: https://inthemiddleofthewhirlwind.wordpress.com/precarious-labor-a-feminist-viewpoint/ [Accessed 30 December 2017].

Feher, M., 2009. Self-Appreciation: Or, the Aspirations of Human Capital. *Public Culture*, 21(1), pp.21–41.

Feldhendler, D., 1994. Augusto Boal and Jacob L. Moreno. In: Mady Schutzman and Jan Cohen-Cruz, eds. *Playing Boal: Theatre, Therapy, Activism*. Routledge, Abingdon, Oxon and New York, pp.87–109.

Fiduccia, J., 2008. Omer Fast: A Multiple 'I'. *Uovo Magazine*, (17), April, pp.156–76.

Fischer-Lichte, E., 2008. *The Transformative Power of Performance: A New Aesthetics*. London: Routledge

Fisher, M., 2009. *Capitalist Realism: Is There No Alternative?* Winchester: Zero Books.

Foster, H. ed., 1983. *The Anti-Aesthetic: Essays on Postmodern Culture*. Port Townsend, Washington: Bay Press.

Foster, H., 1996a. Obscene, Abject, Traumatic. *October*, 78, pp.106–24.

Foster, H., 1996b. *The Return of the Real: The Avant-Garde at the End of the Century*. Cambridge, MA, London: MIT Press (October books.

Foster, H., 2004. Arty Party. In: *London Review of Books*. London: Nicholas Spice, pp.21–2.

Foster, H., 2006. Chat Rooms (2004). In: C. Bishop, ed. *Participation*, Documents of Contemporary Art. London and Cambridge, MA: Whitechapel and MIT Press. pp.190–5.

Foster, H., 2015. *Bad New Days: Art, Criticism, Emergency*. London and New York: Verso Books.

Foucault, M., 1984. Truth and Power: An Interview with A. Fontana and P. Pasquino. In: P. Rabinow, ed. *The Foucault Reader*. New York: Pantheon. pp.51–75.

Foucault, M., 1985. *Discourse and Truth: The Problematization of Parrhesia. 6 Lectures Given by Michel Foucault at the University of California at Berkeley, Oct–Nov. 1983*. [online] foucault.info. Available at: http://www.foucault.info/system/files/pdf/DiscourseAndTruth_MichelFoucault_1983_0.pdf [Accessed 6 June 2017].

Foucault, M., 2011. *The Courage of the Truth (The Government of Self and Others II): Lectures at the Collège de France 1983–1984*. Translated by G. Burchell. Basingstoke and New York: Palgrave Macmillan.

Fowler, C., 2013. Once More with Feeling: Performing the Self in the Work of Gillian Wearing, Kutluğ Ataman and Phil Collins. *Moving Image Review & Art Journal*, 2(1), pp.10–24.

Fox, O., 2018. *Performance Art Can Change Your Life! Shame Attacking and Parrhesia as Feminist Practices of Freedom*. Unpublished PhD thesis. Goldsmiths University.

Fraser, N., 2013. *Fortunes of Feminism: From State-Managed Capitalism to Neoliberal Crisis*. London and Brooklyn, NY: Verso Books.

French, R. and Simpson, P., 2010. The 'Work Group': Redressing the Balance in Bion's Experiences in Groups. *Human Relations*, 63(12), pp.1859–78.

Froggatt, W., 2005. *A Brief Introduction to Rational Emotive Behaviour Therapy*. Available at: https://www.researchgate.net/publication/237435902_Rational_Emotive_Behaviour_Therapy [Accessed 12 June 2017].

Furedi, F., 2004. *Therapy Culture: Cultivating Vulnerability in an Uncertain Age*. London: Routledge.

Genosko, G., 2000. The Life and Work of Félix Guattari: From Transversality to Ecosophy. In: *The Three Ecologies*. Translated by Ian Pindar and Paul Sutton. London and Brunswick, NJ: The Athlone Press. pp.106–60.

Gill, R., 2008. Culture and Subjectivity in Neoliberal and Postfeminist Times. *Subjectivity*, 25, pp.432–45.

Gill, R. and Pratt, A., 2008. In the Social Factory? Immaterial Labour, Precariousness and Cultural Work. *Theory, Culture & Society*, 25(7–8), pp.1–30.

Gilligan, M., 2007. The Beggar's Pantomime: Melanie Gilligan on Performance and Its Appropriations. *Artforum*, 45(10), pp.426–33.

Gilligan, M., 2008. *Crisis in the Credit System*. [online] Artangel. Available at: https://www.artangel.org.uk/project/crisis-in-the-credit-system/ [Accessed 6 March 2010].

Gilligan, M., and Vishmidt, M., 2018. Economic Subjectivities and Crisis. Available at: http://theartistsinstitute.org/wp-content/uploads/2018/02/Economic_Subjectivities_and_Crisis.pdf, [Accessed 24 October 2019].

Goffey, A., 2016. Guattari and Transversality: Institutions, Analysis and Experimentation. *Radical Philosophy*, 195, pp.38–47.

Gogarty, L.A., 2017. 'Usefulness' in Contemporary Art and Politics. *Third Text*, 31(1), pp.117–32.

Gonçalves, R., Pedrozo, A.L., Freire Coutinho, E.S., Figueira, I. and Ventura, P., 2012. *Efficacy of Virtual Reality Exposure Therapy in the Treatment of PTSD: A Systematic Review*. [online] PLoS ONE. Available at: https://www.ncbi.nlm.nih.gov/pmc/articles/PMC3531396/.

Grusin, R.A., 2010. *Premediation: Affect and Mediality after 9/11*. Basingstoke: Palgrave Macmillan.

Guattari, F., 1995. *Chaosmosis: An Ethico-Aesthetic Paradigm*. Translated by P. Bains. and Translated by J. Pefanis. Bloomington and Indianapolis: Indiana University Press.

Guattari, F., 2000. *The Three Ecologies*. Translated by I. Pindar. and Translated by P. Sutton. London and Brunswick, NJ: The Athlone Press.

Guattari, F., 2009. *Chaosophy: Texts and Interviews, 1972–1977*. S. Lotringer, ed. Translated by D.L. Sweet, J. Becker and T. Adkins. Los Angeles, CA: Semiotext(e).

Guattari, F., 2011. *The Machinic Unconscious: Essays in Schizoanalysis*. Translated by T. Adkins. Los Angeles, CA: Semiotext(e).

Guattari, F., 2015. *Psychoanalysis and Transversality: Texts and Interviews 1955–1971*. Translated by A. Hodges. Los Angeles, CA: Semiotext(e).

Guattari, F. and Rolnik, S., 2008. *Molecular Revolution in Brazil*. Translated by B. Holmes. and Translated by K. Clapshow. Los Angeles, CA: Semiotext(e) (Semiotext(e) foreign agents).

Guattari, F. and Zahm, O., 2011. On Contemporary Art: Interview with Oliver Zahm, April 1992. In: E. Alliez and A. Goffey, eds. *The Guattari Effect*. London and New York: Continuum. pp.40–53.

Halpern, S., 2008. Virtual Iraq: Using Simulation to Treat a New Generation of Traumatized Veterans. *The New Yorker*. [online] 19 May. Available at: https://www.newyorker.com/magazine/2008/05/19/virtual-iraq.

Han, B.-C., 2015. *The Burnout Society*. Translated by E. Butler. Stanford, CA: Stanford University Press.

Hanafin, R., 2010. *Virtual Reality Combat Simulations as a Treatment for PTSD*. [online] Veterans Today. Available at: https://www.veteranstodayarchives.com/2010/05/18/dr-sally-satel-promotes-virtual-reality-war-games-as-a-treatment-for-ptsd/.

Hansen, M.B., 2004. Room-for-Play: Benjamin's Gamble with Cinema. *October*, 109, pp.3–45.

Hansen, M.B.N., 2006. *Bodies in Code: Interfaces with Digital Media*. New York, London: Routledge.

Hansen, M.B.N., 2012. Technics beyond the Temporal Object. *New Formations*, 77, pp.44–62.

Hansen, M.B.N., 2015. *Feed-forward: On the Future of Twenty-First-Century Media*. Chicago: The University of Chicago Press.

Haraway, D.J., 1988. Situated Knowledges: The Science Question in Feminism and the Privilege of Partial Perspective. *Feminist Studies*, 14(3), pp.575–99.

Haraway, D.J., 1991. *Simians, Cyborgs and Women: The Reinvention of Nature*. London: Free Association.

Harbord, J., 2007. *The Evolution of Film: Rethinking Film Studies*. Cambridge, UK, Malden, MA: Polity.

Hardt, M. and Negri, A., 2001. *Empire*. Cambridge, MA and London: Harvard University Press.

Hess, E. and Jokeit, H., 2010. *Neurocapitalism*. [online] Open Democracy. Available at: https://www.opendemocracy.net/en/neurocapitalism [Accessed 6 June 2018].

Hevda, J., n.d. *Sick Woman Theory*. [online] Mask Magazine. Available at: http://www.maskmagazine.com/not-again/struggle/sick-woman-theory [Accessed 22 March 2018].

Hirsch, A., 2016. gURLS Performance Text. Available at: http://therealannhirsch.com/writing/gurls/ [Accessed 6 June 2017].

Holert, T., 2012. Subjects of Finance: Melanie Gilligan Interviewed by Tom Holert. *Grey Room*, 46, pp.84–99.

Holl, U., 2014. Farocki's Cinematic Historiography: Reconstructing the Visible. *e-flux*, [online] 59. Available at: https://www.e-flux.com/journal/59/61118/farocki-s-cinematic-historiography-reconstructing-the-visible/ [Accessed 22 June 2017].

Horning, R., 2013. *Games of Truth*. [online] The New Inquiry. Available at: https://thenewinquiry.com/blog/games-of-truth/.

Illouz, E., 2007. *Cold Intimacies: The Making of Emotional Capitalism*. Cambridge: Polity.

Illouz, E., 2008. *Saving the Modern Soul: Therapy, Emotions, and the Culture of Self-Help*. Berkeley and Los Angeles, CA and London: University of California Press.

Indrisek, S., 2011. Boundary Issues. *Modern Painters*, 23(1), February, pp.46–51.

Jones, A., 2006. *Self/Image: Technology, Representation, and the Contemporary Subject*. London: Routledge.

Kester, G.H., 1997. Aesthetics after the End of Art: An Interview with Susan Buck-Morss. *Art Journal*, 56 (1), pp.38–45.

Kiefer, A. and Laser, L.M., 2016. Angie Keefer and Liz Magic Laser. *BOMB*, (138), pp.76–86.

Kisner, J., 2017. The Politics of Conspicuous Displays of Self-Care. *The New Yorker*. [online] 14 March. Available at: https://www.newyorker.com/culture/culture-desk/the-politics-of-selfcare [Accessed 1 October 2017].

Kotz, L., 1992. The Body You Want: Liz Kotz Interviews Judith Butler. *Artforum*, November, pp.82–9.

Kraus, C., 2015. Leigh Ledare by Chris Kraus. *Bomb*, 132, pp.56–64.

Kuhn, A. ed., 2013. *Little Madnesses: Winnicott, Transitional Phenomena and Cultural Experience*. London and New York: I.B. Tauris.

Lacan, J., [1966] 1977. The Function and Field of Speech and Language in Psychoanalysis. In *Écrits: A Selection*. Translated by Alan Sheridan. London: Tavistock; New York: W.W. Norton. pp.30–113.

Laplanche, J., 1999. *Essays on Otherness*. London and New York: Routledge.

Laser, L.M., n.d. *New York CLose Up: Liz Magic Laser Feeeeeeels Your Pain*. Art21. 29 June 2012. Available at: https://www.youtube.com/watch?v=31Vr6F47fGc [Accessed March 2017].

Latour, B., 2005. *Reassembling the Social: An Introduction to Actor-Network-Theory*. Clarendon Lectures in Management Studies. Oxford and New York: Oxford University Press.

Lazzarato, M., 2014a. *Signs and Machines: Capitalism and the production of subjectivity*. Translated by J.D. Jordan. Los Angeles, CA: Semiotext(e).

Lazzarato, M., 2014b. Does Cognitive Capitalism Exist? In: W. Neidich, ed. *Psychopathologies of Cogntive Capitalism: Part Two*. Berlin: Archive Books. pp.93–112.

Lemke, T., 2001. 'The Birth of Bio-politics': Michel Foucault's Lecture at the Collège de France on Neo-liberal Governmentality. *Economy and Society*, 30(2), pp.190–207.

Lemmens, P., 2011. 'This System Does Not Produce Pleasure Anymore': An Interview with Bernard Stiegler. *Krisis: Journal for Contemporary Philosophy*, (1), pp.33–41.

Leven, B., 2012. The Forgetting of Aesthetics: Individuation, Technology, and Aesthetics in the Work of Bernard Stiegler. *New Formations*, 77, pp.76–96.

Levin, L., 2009. The Performative Force of Photography. *Photography and Culture*, 2(3), pp.327–36.

Leys, R., 2000. *Trauma: A Genealogy*. Chicago and London: The University of Chicago Press.

Leys, R., 2017. *The Ascent of Affect: Genealogy and Critique*. Chicago and London: The University of Chicago Press.

Lorde, A., 1988. *A Burst of Light*. Ithaca, NY: Firebrand Books.

Lu, S., 2013. *Antagonistic Therapy – Krzysztof Wodiczko's 'Abraham Lincoln: War Veteran Projection'*. [unpublished dissertation] University of Pittsburgh. Available at: https://nyu.academia.edu/SiqiaoLu [Accessed 7 May 2018].

Lütticken, S., 2005. An Arena in Which to Reenact. In: Sven Lutticken, ed. *Life, Once More: Forms of Reenactment in Contemporary Art*. Netherlands: Witte de With Center for Contemporary Art. pp.17–60.

Lydén, K., 2014. Therapy for a Pathological Capitalism. In: W. Neidich, ed. *The Psychopathologies of Cognitive Capitalism: Part Two*. Berlin: Archive Books. pp.113–31.

Madsen, O.J., 2014. *The Therapeutic Turn: How Psychology Altered Western Culture*. New York and Hove: Routledge.

Magagnoli, P., 2013. Capitalism as Creative Destruction: The Representation of the Economic Crisis in Hito Steyerl's 'In Free Fall'. *Third Text*, 27(6), pp.723–34.

Mahdawi, A., 2017. Generation Treat Yo' Self: The Problem with 'Self-care'. *The Guardian*. [online] 12 January. Available at: https://www.theguardian.com/lifeandstyle/2017/jan/12/self-care-problems-solange-knowles [Accessed 1 October 2017].

Malabou, C., 2012. *The New Wounded: From Neurosis to Brain Damage*. New York: Fordham University Press (Forms of living).

Mannoni, [1969] 2003. I Know Well, but All the Same. In: M.A. Rothenberg, D.A. Foster, and S. Žižek, eds. *Perversion and the Social Relation*. Durham, NC: Duke University Press. pp. 68–92.

Markham, T., 2019. Affective Solidarity and Mediated Distant Suffering: In Defence of Mere Feltness. *International Journal of Cultural Studies*, 22(4), pp.467–80.

Martin, R., 2013. Inhabiting the Image: Photography, Therapy and Re-enactment Phototherapy. In: D. Loewenthal, ed. *Phototherapy and Therapeutic Photography in a Digital Age*. London and New York: Routledge. pp.69–81.

Martin, R. and Spence, J., 1985. New Portraits for Old: The Use of the Camera in Therapy. *Feminist Review*, (Spring 19), pp.66–75.

McCoy, A., 2014. *In Conversation: Krysztof Wodiczko with Ann McCoy*. [online] The Brooklyn Rail: Critical Perspectives on Arts, Politics, and Culture. Available at: https://brooklynrail.org/2014/02/art/krzysztof-wodiczko-with-ann-mccoy [Accessed 3 March 2017].

Mitchell, J., 2005. Theory as an Object. *October*, 113(Summer), pp.27–38.

Molesworth, H., 2018. *Art Is Medicine*. New York: Artforum. pp.164, 166–8, 170.

Moulier Boutang, Y., 2011. *Cognitive Capitalism*. Translated by E. Emery. Cambridge, UK and Malden, MA: Polity Press.

Mueller, R., 1989. *Bertolt Brecht and the Theory of Media*. Lincoln and London: University of Nebraska Press.

Mulvey, M., January 2009. Is There Sincerity in Hollow Speech? Feeling the Cliche in Contemporary Performance. *NOWISWHERE Contemporary Art Magazine*. London. pp.16–21.

Niessen, N., 2018. 'Mad Men' and Mindfulness. *Discourse*, 40(3), pp.273–307.

Nijdam, M.J. and Vermetten, E., 2018. Moving Forward in Treatment of Posttraumatic Stress Disorder: Innovations to Exposure-based Therapy. *European Journal of Psychotraumatology*, [online] 9(1). Available at: https://www.ncbi.nlm.nih.gov/pmc/articles/PMC5965022/ [Accessed 6 January 2019].

Nolan, J.L., 1998. *The Therapeutic State: Justifying Government at Century's End*. NewYork: New York University Press.

Nunes, S., 2015. *In Conversation with Selected 5 Artist Lucy Beech*. [online] Available at: http://www.fact.co.uk/news-articles/2015/06/in-conversation-with-selected-5-artist-lucy-beech.aspx [Accessed 30 December 2017].

Pantenburg, V., 2016. 'Now that's Brecht at last!': Harun Farocki's Observational Films. In: E. Balsom and H. Peleg, eds. *Documentary Across Disciplines*. Berlin and Cambridge, MA and London: Haus der Kulturen der Welt and MIT Press. pp.142–63.

Parker, A. and Sedgwick, E.K., 1995. *Performativity and Performance*. London and New York: Routledge.

Patierno, M., Jhally, S. and Hirshorn, H. eds., 1997. *bell hooks—Cultural Criticism & Transformation*. Available at: https://www.mediaed.org/transcripts/Bell-Hooks-Transcript.pdf [Accessed 6 June 2019].

Pearlman, S., Seth-Smith, F., Treneman, M. and Gorney, C., 2013. Seeing Is Believing. *Context*, (February), pp.22–5.

Pisters, P., 2012. *The Neuro-Image: A Deleuzian Film-Philosophy of Digital Screen Culture*. Stanford, CA: Stanford University Press.

Pisters, P., 2017. Orchestration of the Senses in Yellow: Eisenstein's Fourth Dimension, Memory, and Mirror-Touch Synaesthesia. In: D. Martin, ed. *Mirror-Touch Synaesthesia: Thresholds of Empathy with Art*. Oxford: Oxford University Press. pp.71–90.

Polack, J.-C., 2011. Analysis, between Psycho and Schizo. In: E. Alliez and A. Goffey, eds. *The Guattari Effect*. London and New York: Continuum. pp.57–67.

Pollock, G., 2013. *After-affects After-Images: Trauma and Aesthetic Transformation in the Virtual Feminist Museum*. Manchester: Manchester University Press.

Prozorov, S., 2017. Foucault's Affirmative Biopolitics: Cynic Parrhesia and the Biopower of the Powerless. *Political Theory*, 45(6), pp.801–23.

Pugh, R., 2016. PlayStation Game Helps Veterans in Prison Deal with Trauma. [online] *The Guardian*. Available at: https://www.theguardian.com/social-care-network/2016/jun/13/playstation-game-ff-gaiden-veterans-prison-fact [Accessed 19 August 2019].

Roelofs, M., 2015. *The Cultural Promise of the Aesthetic*. London and New York: Bloomsbury.

Rose, N.S., 1998. *Inventing Our Selves: Psychology, Power and Personhood*. Cambridge: Cambridge University Press.

Ross, D., 2007. Politics, Terror, and Traumatypical Imagery. In: M. Sharpe, M. Noonan and J. Freddi, eds. *Trauma, History, Philosophy*. Newcastle: Cambridge Scholars Publishing. pp.230–46.

Rottenberg, C., 2018. *The Rise of Neoliberal Feminism*. New York: Oxford University Press.

Rowbotham, S., 2008. Jolting Memory: 'Nightcleaners' Recalled. In: M. Ruido, ed. *Plan Rosebud: On Images, Sites and Politics of Memory*. Santiago de Compostela: CGAC. p.13.

Russo, R.L., 2010. *Videoinsight®: Healing with Contemporary Art*. In: Biblioteca d'arte contemporanea. Milan: Silvana Editoriale.

Scepanski, K. ed., 2014. *Liz Magic Laser Public Relations/ Öffentlichkeitsarbeit*. Berlin: Sternberg Press.

Schutzman, M., 1994. Brechtian Shamanism. In: Mady Schutzman and Jan Cohen-Cruz, eds. *Playing Boal: Theatre, Therapy, Activism*. Oxon and New York: Routledge, Abingdon. pp.137–55.

Schutzman, M., Cohen-Cruz, J. eds., 1994. Playing Boal: Theatre, Therapy, Activism. Oxon and New York: Routledge, Abingdon.

Sedgwick, E.K., 2003. *Touching Feeling: Affect, Pedagogy, Performativity*. Durham, North Carolina: Duke University Press.

Seem, M.D., 1974. Interview: Felix Guattari. *Diacritics*, 4(3), pp.38–41.

Seltzer, M., 1997. Wound Culture: Trauma in the Pathological Public Sphere. *October*, 80, pp.3–26.

Shapiro, E.R. and Carr, A.W., 2012. An Introduction to Tavistock-Style Group Relations Conference Learning. *Organisational and Social Dynamics*, 12(1), pp.70–80.

Shaviro, S., 2010. *Post Cinematic Affect*. Winchester: Zero Books.

Shaviro, S., 2015. *No Speed Limit: Three Essays on Accelerationism*. Minneapolis: University of Minnesota Press.

Sheffield Doc Fest, 2018. *The Task + Extended Q&A*. [online] Available at: https://ly.yes-vlip.lv/video/%2FPYcsYQAXHEy%2Bmo%3D.html [Accessed 6 January 2019].

Sillars, L. ed., 2015. *Omer Fast: Present Continuous*. Gateshead, England: Baltic Center for Contemporary Art.

Simblist, N., 2012. Interview: Omer Fast.... *might be good*, [online] (195), 27 July. Available at: http://www.fluentcollab.org/mbg/index.php/interview/index/195/134 [Accessed 3 March 2014].

Smith, J., 2013. Soul on Strike. In: W. Neidich and A. De Boever, eds. *The Psychopathologies of Cognitive Capitalism: Part One*. Berlin: Archive Books. pp.33–44.

Spivak, G.C., 1988. Can the Subaltern Speak? In: C. Nelson and L. Grossberg, eds. *Marxism and the Interpretation of Culture*. London: Macmillan. pp.271–313.

Steffen, P., 2011. Liz Magic Laser. *Flash Art*, p.105.

Steyerl, H., 2012. *The Wretched of the Screen*. Berlin, Germany: Sternberg Press.

Stiegler, B., 2009. *Technics and Time 2: Disorientation*. Translated by S. Barker. Stanford: Stanford University Press.

Stiegler, B., 2011a. Suffocated Desire, or How the Cultural Industry Destroys the Individual: Contribution to a Theory of Mass Consumption. Translated by J. Rossouw. *Parrhesia*, 13, pp.52–61.

Stiegler, B., 2011b. *Technics and Time*. Translated by S.F. Barker. Stanford, CA: Stanford University Press.

Stiegler, B., 2012. Care Within the Limits of Capitalism, Economizing Means Taking Care. In: T. Cohen, ed. *Telemorphosis Theory in the Era of Climate Change*. pp.104–20. Available at: http://openhumanitiespress.org/books/download/Cohen_2012_Telemorphosis.pdf [Accessed 6 June 2018].

Stiegler, B., 2013a. *What Makes Life Worth Living: On Pharmacology*. Translated by D. Ross. Cambridge, UK: Polity.

Stiegler, B., 2013b. Organology of Dreams and Archi-Cinema. Translated by D. Ross. *Screening the Past*, [online] (36). Available at: http://www.screeningthepast.com/2013/06/the-organology-of-dreams-and-arche-cinema/ [Accessed 7 December 2017].

Stiegler, B., 2014. *Symbolic Misery. Volume 1: The Hyper-Industrial Epoch*. Translated by B. Norman. Cambridge, England: Polity Press.

Taylor, C., 1991. *The Ethics of Authenticity*. Cambridge, Massachusetts: London, England: Harvard University Press.

Taylor, D., 2003. *The Archive and the Repertoire: Performing Cultural Memory in the Americas*. Durham and London: Duke University Press.

Ten Brink, J. and Oppenheimer, J. eds., 2012. *Killer Images: Documentary Film, Memory and the Performance of Violence*. New York and Chicester West Sussex: Columbia University Press.

Terranova, T., 2013. Ordinary Psychopathologies of Cognitive Capitalism. In: A. De Boever and W. Neidich, eds. *The Psychopathologies of Cognitive Capitalism: Part One*. Berlin: Archive Books. pp.45–68.

Toscano, A. and Kinkle, J., 2015. *Cartographies of the Absolute*. Winchester: Zero Books.

Totschnig, W., 2017. Arendt's Notion of Natality: An Attempt at Clarification. *Ideas y Valores*, 66(165), pp.327–46.

Trilling, L., 1972. *Sincerity and Authenticity*. Cambridge, MA: Harvard University Press.

Troeller, J., 2014. The Factographic Gesture. In: K. Scepanski, ed. *Liz Magic Laser: Public Relations/ Offentlichkeitsarbeit*. Berlin: Sternberg Press. pp.118–25.

Väliaho, P., 2014. *Biopolitical Screens: Image, Power, and the Neoliberal Brain*. Cambridge, MA: MIT Press (Leonardo).

Verhagen, M., 2009. Pleasure and Pain: Omer Fast interviewed by Marcus Verhagen. *Art Monthly*, (330), October, pp.1–4.

Vinyes Albes, M., 2015. Interview: 'Present Continuous' with Omer Fast. In: L. Sillars, ed. *Omer Fast: Present Continuous*. Gateshead: Baltic Center for Contemporary Art.

Vishmidt, M., 2013. *Permanent Reproductive Crisis: An Interview with Silvia Federici*. [online] Mute. Available at: http://www.metamute.org/editorial/

articles/permanent-reproductive-crisis-interview-silvia-federici#sdfootnote1anc [Accessed 30 December 2017].

Voela, A. and Rothschild, L., 2019. Creative Failure: Stiegler, Psychoanalysis and the Promise of a Life Worth Living. *New Formations*, (95), pp.54–69.

Waller, M.A., 2011. Mark Aerial Waller Interviews Carry Gorney. Available at: http://www.markaerialwaller.com/Interview%20with%20carry%20gorney.html [Accessed 20 June 2017].

Walsh, M., 2015. Performing Resistance to Performing Autonomy and Back Again: Alex Bag Meets Ann Hirsch. *MIRAJ: Moving Image Review and Art Journal*, 4(1 & 2), pp.13–41.

Walsh, M. 2016. Archiving Loss in the Green Backyard: Jessie Brennan's Recollection-objects. In: *Re: development: Voices, Cyanotypes & Writings from the Green Backyard*. London: Silent Grid. pp.88–90.

Walsh, M., 2019. Female Solidarity as Uncommodified Value: Lucy Beech's Cannibals and Rehana Zaman's Some Women, Other Women and All the Bittermen. In: L. Reynolds, ed. *Women Artists, Feminism and Film*. London and New York: Bloomsbury. pp.229–43.

War, Trauma and Public Art: A Panel with Krzysztof Wodiczko, Ani Buk, Rosalyn Deutsche, Joseph Ledoux, Carl Cannon and Carol Becker. n.d. Directed by More Art and NYU. Available at: https://vimeo.com/92063206.

Waxman, L., 2017. Leigh Ledare at the Art Institute of Chicago. *Chicago Tribune*. Available at: https://www.tribpub.com/gdpr/chicagotribune.com/ [Accessed 3 December 2017].

Wearing, G., 2012. *Gillian Wearing*. London: Whitechapel Gallery, Ridinghouse, Kunstsammlung Nordhein-Westfalen.

Williams, A. and Srnicek, N., 2013. *#Accelerate: Manifesto for an Accelerationist Politics*. [Blog] Critical Legal Thinking. Available at: http://criticallegalthinking.com/2013/05/14/accelerate-manifesto-for-an-accelerationist-politics/ [Accessed 6 December 2016].

Williams, T., 2014. Street Scenes. In: K. Scepanski, ed. *Liz Magic Laser: Public Relations/ Offentlichkeitsarbeit*. Berlin: Sternberg Press. pp.126–34.

Wilson, E.A., 2015. *Gut Feminism*. In: Next Wave: New Directions in Women's Studies. Durham and London: Duke University Press.

Winnicott, D.W., 1953. Transitional Objects and Transitional Phenomena: A Study of the First Not-Me Possession. *The International Journal of Psychoanalysis*, 34, pp.89–97.

Winnicott, D.W., 1974. Fear of Breakdown. *International Review of Psychoanalysis*, 1, pp.103–7.

Winnicott, D.W., [1971] 2001. *Playing and Reality*. London: Brunner-Routledge.

Yates, C., 2014. Psychoanalysis and Television: Notes towards a psycho-cultural approach. In: C. Bainbridge, I. Ward and C. Yates, eds. *Television and Psychaonalysis: Psycho-cultural Perspectives*, Psychoanalysis and Popular Culture. London: Karnac Books. pp.1–30.

Zaman, R. and Guy, L., 2015. *Mindless Culture, Unskilled Labour: A Conversation*. [online] Available at: http://wheresleft y.tumblr.com/post/121107183546/mindless-culture-unskilled-labour-a-conversation.

Zechner, M. and Rübner Hansen, B., 2012. Unchained Melodies of the New Proletariat: A Review of For a New Critique of Political Economy. *Generation*. [online] 2 October. Available at: http://www.generation-online.org/other/stieglerreview.htm [Accessed 6 December 2016].

Zepke, S., 2012. Art and the Aesthetics of the Interface; Autonomy, Sensation and Biopolitics. In: R. Braidotti and P. Pisters, eds. *Revisiting Normativity with Deleuze*. London and New York: Bloomsbury. pp.218–32.

Index

Abraham Lincoln: War Veteran Projection 11, 47, 56–8
Achiampong, Larry and David Blandy 44
achievement society 13, 132, 172–3
actants 107, 111, 196 n.1; social actors 33
adaptation, in Berardi 100–1; in Stiegler 122, 155
adoption, in Stiegler 122
Adorno, Theodor and Max Horkheimer 21
aesthetic inefficacy 88, 93, 95, 104
aesthetics 1, 5, 14, 181, 185 n.2, 187 n.7; accelerationist 63, 88; in Berardi 151; in Guattari 77, 186 n.15; pharmacological 2–3, 46, 47, 56, 65, 93, 125, 138; relational 12, 112; in Shaviro 47, 88, 104; in Stiegler 23–4, therapeutic 9, 15, 20, 173, 178
affective 5, 10, 67, 70, 79, 154, 191 n.16; labour 152–3
affectsphere 95, 184
agency 32, 107, 119, 152
Ahmad, Ayesha 66
Ahmed, Sara 58, 94
anamnesic 22
anti-aesthetic 5
Anti-Oedipus: Capitalism and Schizophrenia 79
anxiety 43, 63, 97, 104, 139, 192 n.16, 192 n.17; *see also* symptoms
apology, performativity of 93; politics of 94; speech act of 94
Arendt, Hannah 85
art therapy 3–4, 14, 56, 58
aspirational selfhood 4, 134; aspirational subjects 129
Austin, J.L. 8, 94, 180, 199 n.12
Autogenic Training 18
Autonomist theories of labour 71, 152

Balsom, Erika 53–4
Bakhtin, Mikhail 159
basic-assumption mentality and functioning 114, 116; *see also* group-work mentality
Baumgarten, Alexander 24
becoming-indigestible 176
Beech, Lucy 13, 14, 151, 153–64, 166, 168, 183, 202 n.6
Begonia, Marisa 168
behabitives 94
Beller, Jonathan 6, 18–21, 187 n.4
Benjamin, Walter 24–5, 64–5, 111, 186 n.13
Bennett, Jill 1, 54
Berardi, Franco 'Bifo' 3, 6, 36, 67–71, 74, 77, 80, 99–102, 104–5, 151–2, 183, 192 n.6, 203 n.2
Berlant, Lauren 10, 14, 173, 182–4
Bernes, Jasper J. 77
Bersani, Leo 59, 184
Billingham, Richard 141
Bion, Wilfred 12, 108, 113–14, 116, 120, 177
biopolitical 32, 73, 75, 78, 80, 136; governance 73, 78, 80, 90
biopolitics 6, 39
biocapitalism 5
Boal, Augusto 144–5, 147, 200 n.27
Boudry, Pauline 175
Bourriaud, Nicolas 112
Brady, Sara 42–4
Braidotti, Rosi 152
Brecht 54, 96, 145, 188 n.1
Brechtian 17, 30, 54; Lehrstücke 165
Brunsdon, Charlotte 165
Buck-Morss, Susan 14, 24–5, 55, 90, 187 n.7
Buried Alive 155, 157, 160–3, 166
Butler, Judith 8–9, 50, 131, 176, 179

Cannibals 155, 157–60, 166, 168–9
capitalism, cognitive 4–6, 20, 26, 36, 67, 69–71, 73–5, 80–1, 129, 134, 137, 151–2, 154–5, 172, 185 n.8; commodity 10; communicative 5; global 25, 50, 59, 88, 158, 164; totalitarian 21, 27
care of the self 137–8, 172, 173
The Casting 11, 48, 50–2, 59, 64
catharsis 58, 101, 144–5, 147; abreactive 97; Aristolean 145
cathartic function 35
CBT, *see* cognitive behavioural therapy
Celis Bueno, Claudio 30, 35
Chamarette, Jenny 148
Chaosophy 80
Charlesworth, Amy 164, 166
The Chittendens 76
Coetzee, J.M. 127–8, 133
cognitive behavioural therapy 43, 129
collective subjectivity 11, 12, 82, 117, 182
The Common Sense 67, 80–2
confabulation 54, 60; *also see* fabulation
Continuity 48
creative destruction 69, 76–7, 193 n.7
Crisis in the Credit System 67–8, 77
Cruel Optimism 174
The Cultural Politics of Emotions 91
cure 1, 7, 10–11, 15, 20, 24, 27, 35, 39, 43–4, 47, 50, 59, 92, 117, 129, 137, 145, 176–7, 184
cynic, the 135–6

The Dangerous Rise of Therapeutic Education 29
Deleuze, Gilles 53, 79
Deleuze, Gilles and Félix Guattari 79, 176
depression 70, 99, 104, 139; *see under* symptoms
Derrida, Jacques 7–8, 21, 179, 198 n.3
deterritorialization 81
dissociation 38, 43, 61, 66, 191 n.16

Ecclestone and Hayes 29, 185 n.5
emotional labour 162
emotional life 15, 131, 134, 139
emotions 72, 92, 134–5, 145, 147, 149; conflictual 98, 141; negative 100, 155, 161–2
empathy 49, 53–4, 58, 101
Engel, Antke and Renate Lorenz 175–6
establishment 32, 117
Excitable Speech 176
exhaustion 99, 104
Experiences in Groups 114, 177
exposure therapy 13, 43, 133–5, 183
exteriority 7, 21, 42

fabulation 13, 49, 64; *also see* confabulation
Farocki, Harun 10–11, 27–39, 41–2, 44, 48, 50, 59, 182, 188 n.2
Fast, Omer 3, 11, 47–51, 53–6, 61–2, 64, 182
fear of breakdown 89, 95
Federici, Silvia 71, 152, 154, 169, 201 n.2
feed-forward structure 111
Feher, Michel 167–8, 203 n.16
feminism, lean in 132, 198 n.8; socialist 164
feminist neoliberal subject 160
FF Gaiden: Control 44–6
5 162–3
5000 Feet Is the Best 11, 48–50, 60–1, 64
Fordism 154, 167
Fortunes of Feminism 169
Foster, Hal 4–5, 112, 134
Foucault, Michel 31, 34, 135–7, 171, 174, 199 n.12
Fox, Oriana 13, 127, 130–3, 138–9, 199 n.13
Fraser, Nancy 169
Full Spectrum Warrior 40
Furedi, Frank 2, 63, 90, 100–11, 134

Genosko, Gary 67, 69, 117
Gilligan, Melanie 11, 67–70, 72, 75–8, 80–2, 85, 117, 182, 192 n.4
Gilligan, Melanie and Marina Vishmidt 76, 79
Goffey, Andrew 32, 117
The Good Story: Exchanges on Truth 127
Gorney, Carry 110–11
group subject 117–18, 125; group subjectivity 116

group-work mentality 114–16, 118–21; *see also* basic-assumption mentality and functioning
Guattari, Félix 6, 13, 15, 32, 68, 77–81, 85, 116–17, 123–5, 188 n.3, 197 n.16, 197 n.17

Han, Byung-Chul 132
Hansen, Miriam Bratu 65
Hansen, Mark B. N. 111
Haraway, Donna 153, 164
Harbord, Janet 59
hermeneutics of suspicion 17
Hirsch, Ann 133–4
homeopathic magic 9, 25–6, 47–8, 63, 87
homeopathic mimicry 9, 12, 47, 63–4, 66–7, 76, 81, 83, 92, 182–4
Horning, Rob 135, 149
How to Live in the FRG 27–30, 32, 35–6
human capital 29, 167, 168, 171
hypnosis 25, 38–9
hypomnesis 7, 127

I Feel Your Pain 90–5, 194 n.2
identicality 97, 103–5, 107
identitarian 14, 79, 107, 109, 139, 179
Illouz, Eva 3, 6, 17, 28, 34, 63, 75, 101, 134–5
immanent critique 17, 27, 30, 33, 35, 88
immaterial labour 6, 11, 14, 71, 151–2, 154, 158, 163–5
Immersion 36, 39–40, 42, 44; *see under Serious Games*
Immersive Infantry Trainer 37
immunity 42, 172
industrial-military-image complex 42
inoculation 11, 47, 67, 186 n.13
institution 32, 117–18
institutional object 116–17, 122
institutional organization 32, 123

Janet, Pierre 38–9
Janov, Arthur 95
J4DW; *see* Justice for Domestic Workers
Justice for Domestic Workers 163–4, 166, 168–9

Kisner, Jordan 174
knowledge-how-to-live 27, 32, 35
Krakow Town Hall 56
Kurtz, Arabella 127–8

La Borde 117
Lakoff, George P. 98, 102
Laplanche, Jean 56
The Large Group (Zurich) 12, 108, 112–13, 116, 118–23, 125
Laser, Magic Liz 12, 87, 90–4, 96, 98, 104, 194 n.2, 195 n.8
Lazard, Carolyn 172, 203 n.3
Lazzarato, Maurizio 30, 80–1, 107, 188 n.3
Ledare, Leigh 12–13, 108, 112–14, 116, 118–23
Leeds Animation Workshop 166–7, 203 n.15
Lefebvre, Henri 183
Leigh, Simone 172, 200 n.22
Leven, Bram 23–4
Leys, Ruth 38, 44, 189 n.12, 189 n.17, 190 n.7
Lorde, Audre 173
Lütticken, Sven 75, 164
Lydén, Karl 137

machinic, assemblages 80–1; enslavement 80
Markham, Tim 33
Martin, Rosy 108–10, 196 n.5
Mahdawi, Arwa 174
Maslow, Abraham 167
Merleau-Ponty, Maurice 111
Method 142, 149
method acting 13, 96, 140, 183
military-industrial-technical complex 36
Mitchell, Juliet 97, 103
mother-environment, the 22, 34, 122
Morgellons disease 155–6
Moulier Boutang, Yann 4
Mueller, Roswitha 30

narcotic insulation 24
natality 85
neoliberal capitalism 2, 5–6, 88, 130, 159, 169, 172
neoliberal cognitive capitalism 20, 99, 135, 153, 169, 174, 192 n.4

neuromobilization 69, 71, 97, 99
No Speed Limit 88
Noys, Benjamin 65, 88

The O Show 13, 128–30, 132, 135, 139, 183
operational images 35, 188 n.2
Oury, Jean 117

Parker, Andrew and Eve Kosofsky Sedgwick 129
parrhesia 136–7
performance 8, 40–1, 76, 90, 94, 96, 123, 128, 130, 135–6, 145, 147–8; psychoanalytical performance 125
performance studies 180
performance-to-camera 120, 178
performative 8, 14, 35, 42, 44, 46, 55–6, 62, 75–6, 94, 109, 127–8, 133, 135, 178–9, 183, 189 n.17, 199 n.12
performativity 8–9, 44, 93, 125, 127, 131, 175, 179–80, 184, 186 n.12
pharmacological 1–3, 21, 44, 47, 63, 65, 90, 97, 107, 111, 122, 125, 173, 183
pharmaka 22, 25, 34
pharmakon 1, 7, 21–3, 87, 93, 176–7, 198 n.1
Pharmakon 155, 157, 202 n.6
photo therapy 108, 196 n.4
Phototherapy 108
Popular Unrest 67, 72–4, 77, 81
Post Cinematic Affect 47, 63
post-Fordism 154
post-Fordist 75–6, 154, 164
post-traumatic stress disorder 3, 11, 15, 36, 38–9, 41, 43, 45–7, 60, 62, 182, 189 n.9, 189 n.11, 189 n.16
Primal Speech 12, 87–90, 95–8, 100–5, 182, 196 n.11
primary perception 42
Prozorov, Sergei 136
psychopathologies 2, 6, 67, 69, 74, 172, 182
psychopower 22–3
PTSD, *see under* post-traumatic stress disorder

rational emotive behavioural therapy 3, 13, 128–9, 131–5, 137, 139, 149
REBT, *see under* rational emotive behavioural therapy
re-enactment 13, 30, 32, 38, 40, 42, 55, 141, 146
relational 95, 199 n.15 remedy 198 n.1; truth 128
relationality 88; aesthetic 171; disturbances of 184
rhythmanalysis 20, 183
rhythms 24, 69, 102; bio- 19–20, 23, 26; machinic 71
Roelofs, Monique 171
reparation 59, 95, 186 n.11
reproduction, sphere of 154, 168; social 164
reproductive labour 152
resistance 5, 9, 20, 26, 71, 77, 80, 139, 151, 152, 166, 174–5, 198 n.17; micro-resistance 6, 21, 68, 181
Rist, Pipilotti 10, 17–20, 23, 163
Rose, Nikolas 9, 32
Rottenberg, Catherine 130, 159, 160
Rumbelow, Sam 13, 129, 140, 142–6

Scandalishious 133, 135
Schindler's List 55
Schumpeter, Joseph 76, 193 n.7
secondary mnemonic retentions 42
Sedgwick, Eve Kosofsky 8, 17, 92–3, 95, 141, 162, 180, 195 n.7
self-actualization 10, 132, 137, 144, 167; -styling 142, 153; -cultivation 171, 181, 183; -appreciation 167–8
self-care 14, 160, 172–5, 177, 181, 184, 200 n.22; #selfcare 173
self-esteem 2, 100, 133, 169
Self Made 13, 128–9, 140–2, 145–6, 148
semiocapitalism 6, 67–70, 152
semiologies, signifying 67, 78, 80–1, 125; presignifying 78
semiotics, mixed 68, 78–83, 85; a-signifying 77–82, 85–6
separation 97, 103–5, 107
Serious Games 11, 27, 36–39, 41–44, 46, 50, 59, 182
shame 94, 133, 135, 141, 161–2
shame-attacking 13, 133, 135–6, 138, 142–3
Sharla Shabana Sojourner Selena 173, 177, 179–80, 182
Shaviro, Steven 6, 11, 25, 47, 63–4, 87–9, 171

shyness 132, 133, 139
Simians, Cyborgs and Women: The Reinvention of Nature 164
simulation 40, 44, 93; virtual simulation 38, 42
singularity 25, 107, 127, 175, 183
Smith, Jason 100–11, 172
soap opera 165
soft montage 41, 189 n.14
Some Women, Other Women and All the Bittermen 163, 166, 168, 202 n.10
spectacle 18–19, 58, 92, 156, 187 n.4; political spectacle 93, 95, 97
spect-actor 145–6, 201 n.27
speech acts 8–9, 13, 91, 124–5, 179
Spence, Jo 108–9
Spielberg's List 55
Stanislavski, Konstantin 96, 128
Steyerl, Hito 193 n.10
Stiegler, Bernard 6, 18, 21–5, 31–5, 42, 74, 107, 122, 155, 177, 189 n.8
Strand, Chick 178
subject-groups 123–4
subjection 14, 27, 30, 80–1, 101, 107, 111, 125, 156; subjectification 30, 32, 152, 182; subjectivation 30, 72, 80–1, 107, 118, 125, 136, 188 n.3
subjugated groups 123–4
Sullivan, Catherine 76
survivance 14, 50, 181–2, 186 n.16
symptoms 11, 42–3, 59, 67, 75, 91, 139, 155–7, 162–3, 173–4, 189 n.9

The Task 12, 108, 112, 114, 116, 119–21, 123
Tavistock Institute 12, 108, 113, 119, 183
Tavistock Method 112–13, 118, 121, 197 n.9
Taylor, Diana 179–80
technics 21–2, 24, 33, 35, 111, 122
technologies, of capture 107, 111; of recording 21–2, 127; of subjectification 32
Terranova, Tiziana 5–6, 185 n.8
tertiary industrial projection 42
Theatre of the Oppressed 144, 200 n.27
Therapeutae, the 137–8
therapeutic emotional style 3, 14, 28, 90, 92, 101, 135
therapeutic turn, the 10, 29
thera-poetry 71
The Thought Leader 90, 93–4
Tomkins, Silvan 162
Totschnig, Wolfhart 85
toxic 22–3, 34, 65, 89, 103, 128, 175–7, 183
Toxic 175–6
transitional object 10, 22–3, 33–4, 64, 103–4, 107, 116–17, 122, 147, 182
Transitional Objects and Transitional Phenomena 22
transitional space 7, 22–3, 33, 43, 45, 55, 60, 65–6, 97, 102–3, 109, 119, 122, 152, 166, 173, 177
transindividual 22
transmission, transgenerational 42; transpersonal 66
transmission of, experience 21–2; knowledge 155
trauma 4, 11, 38–9, 42–3, 45, 48–50, 54–6, 62–3, 66, 109, 120, 129, 134, 139, 179, 189 n.8, 189 n.17, 190 n.9, 192 n.17; war trauma 47
trauma-turned-drama 53, 59
Troeller, Jordan 92
truth, -telling 54, 127, 135–6; internal 127; fictional 127, 133, 142; -effects 128, 130, 133–4, 142, 199 n.12

uncommodified, pleasure 154, 166; value 167–8
unconscious 5, 19–20, 39, 44, 56, 92; machinic 79, 193 n.10; optical 111, 114
unconscious identification 12, 103
Until the End of the World 18, 20

Väliaho, Pasi 39, 42, 50
Virno, Paolo 76, 152
Virtual Reality Exposure Therapy 38–9, 41–3
Vishmidt, Marina 70
VRET, *see under* Virtual Reality Exposure Therapy

Waxman, Lori 123
Wenders, Wim 18–21
What Makes Life Worth Living 6, 21, 24, 155, 198 n.1

Wilson, Elizabeth 7, 15, 186 n.11
Winnicott, Donald Woods 6–7, 10, 12, 21–3, 33–5, 65, 89, 95, 97, 102–3, 107, 116, 147
well-being 2, 12–14, 34, 129, 132, 160, 162, 183, 185 n.5, 202 n.6
Women Talking 110
Wearing, Gillian 13, 127–8, 140–1, 146, 148, 200 n.25
Well Being 155, 157, 160, 166
withdrawal 12, 69, 71, 99, 104, 151, 163
Wodiczko, Kryzstof 11, 47, 56–9
Worry Will Vanish Horizon 17, 19–20, 163

Zaman, Rehana 13–14, 151, 153–4, 162–8, 173, 177–8, 183, 201 n.2, 202 n.10, 203 n.13
Zechner, Manuela and Rübner Hansen 153
Žižek, Slavoj 101

Printed by Libri Plureos GmbH in Hamburg,
Germany